Men's
Health
ADVISOR
1992

Men's
Health
ADVISOR
1992

Edited by Michael Lafavore,
Men's Health **Magazine**

 Rodale Press, Emmaus, Pennsylvania

If you have any questions or comments concerning this book, please write: Rodale Press, Book Readers' Service, 33 East Minor Street, Emmaus, PA 18098.

"In Earnest Pain" excerpted from *The Intellectuals* by Paul Johnson. Copyright © 1989 by Paul Johnson. Reprinted by permission of HarperCollins Publishers.

"Fatherly Ways" excerpted from *Staying the Course* by Robert S. Weiss. Copyright © 1990 by Robert S. Weiss. Reprinted with permission of The Free Press, a division of Macmillan, Inc.

"Men Need Men" excerpted from *To Be a Man* by Sam Keen, edited by Keith Thompson. Copyright © 1991 by Keith Thompson. Reprinted with special permission from Jeremy P. Tarcher, Inc., Los Angeles.

"Rational about Money" excerpted from *If I Think about Money So Much, Why Can't I Figure It Out?* by Arlene Modica Matthews. Copyright © 1991 by Arlene Modica Matthews. Reprinted by permission of Summit Books, a division of Simon & Schuster, Inc.

"Rules of the Road" excerpted from *A Life on the Road* by Charles Kuralt. Copyright © 1990 by Charles Kuralt. Reprinted by permission of The Putnam Publishing Group.

"Special Treatment" excerpted from *Love and Profit* by James A. Autry. Copyright © 1991 by James A. Autry. Reprinted with permission of William Morrow and Company, Inc./Publishers, New York.

"A (Very) Short History of the Penis" excerpted from *Facts and Phalluses* by Alexandra Parsons. Copyright © 1989 by Alexandra Parsons. Reprinted with special permission from St. Martin's Press, Inc., New York.

"Watching the Leaves Fall" excerpted from *Downshifting: Reinventing Success on a Slower Track* by Amy Saltzman. Copyright © 1991 by Amy Saltzman. Reprinted by permission of HarperCollins Publishers.

"What Can I Do about My Thinning Hair?" excerpted from *Men's Hair* by George Roberson, with Leonard McGill and Carol Tonsing. Copyright © 1985 by George Roberson. Reprinted with permission of Rawson Associates, an imprint of Macmillan Publishing Company.

ISBN 0–87596–113–4 hardcover
ISSN 1060–9407

2 4 6 8 10 9 7 5 3   hardcover

Contributors to
Men's Health Advisor 1992

PROJECT MANAGER: Russell Wild

PRODUCTION EDITOR: Jane Sherman

COPY EDITOR: Susan G. Berg

COVER DESIGNER: Greg Imhoff

BOOK DESIGNER: Alfred Zelcer

ILLUSTRATOR: Doug Taylor

SECRETARY: Mary Lou Stephen

EXECUTIVE EDITOR, *Men's Health* magazine:
Michael Lafavore

EDITORIAL DIRECTOR: Mark Bricklin

MANAGING EDITOR: Steven Slon

RESEARCH EDITOR: Mary Brophy

OFFICE MANAGER: Susan Campbell

CONTENTS

8 LOOKING GOOD

HAIR CARE 101 ....**189**

If shinier, cleaner, healthier hair is what you're after, read this chapter. Let the experts teach you a thing or two about good-looking locks.

FILL 'ER UP **195**

Smile. When it comes to fixing cavities, picking the right fillin' isn't so chillin'. Here's some helpful information to chew on.

SMOOTH STROKES **197**

Avoiding razor nicks is a matter of sharp skills. Tape these tips on your bathroom mirror.

HIDE YOUR HIDE **200**

Who says there's no effortless way to slim down? Choosing the right wardrobe can make you look 10 pounds lighter.

9 BOD LIKE A ROCK

MAKE GAINS FAST **204**

Get the ultimate workout in just 40 minutes. Dozens of top exercise experts tell you how to squeeze the most pump into the least amount of time.

HOME SWEAT HOME **215**

Why join a health club? A great home gym can be yours for less than you may think. Start your shopping here.

EVEN THOUGH THE SOUND OF IT IS SOMETHING QUITE ATROCIOUS **220**

Super calisthenics aren't so awful. Jumping jacks, push-ups, and crunches are coming back.

STEP UP IN LIFE **224**

There must be a reason stair-climbing machines continue to climb in popularity. Here it is: You can burn 2,000 calories in three 30-minute workouts a week.

WORKOUT TIPS FROM THE PROS **226**

These guys know how to exercise efficiently and safely. Take a few hints from Pat Croce, physical conditioning coach for the Philadelphia Flyers and 76ers, and others.

Introduction

B E Y O N D
B E E R
A N D   S E X

When we first decided to do *Men's Health Advisor,* I asked Russ Wild, a book editor here at Rodale Press, to help me put together a logical outline for the book. He in turn conferred with a female colleague, who insisted that a book written for men need have only two chapters: Beer and Sex. "For what else (hee hee) do men care about?"

As it turns out, plenty. At the request of *Men's Health,* Louis Harris & Associates recently polled a cross section of American men on what they see as essential to their lives. Guess what? Beer wasn't anywhere on the list. And sex rated a mere *sixth.* Here's the list Harris came up with, in order of importance:

1. A happy family
2. A clean, healthy environment
3. Close friends
4. A good income
5. Career success
6. A satisfying sex life

At *Men's Health* we've always taken the word *health* to mean all the things that go with physical heartiness, including family life and friendships, rewarding vacations, a sound environment, and satisfying careers. That's why Russ and I have included readings on all of these subjects in the pages that follow. What about beer and sex? Yeah, you can read about those here, too.

We hope you enjoy this book as much as we enjoyed putting it together. As editors, we oversee the articles that are assembled for each issue of *Men's Health* and for this book. But ultimately, it's the dedicated health writers we have to thank for going out there and finding the stories you'll see here. Here's to all of them—and to you.

To your health!

MICHAEL LAFAVORE
EXECUTIVE EDITOR
Men's Health magazine

Part 1

HOW A MAN STAYS YOUNG

Shooting for 100

No one can guarantee that you'll live to be 100 years old—but the odds are better than ever. Here's a primer on how to increase your odds.

• • • • • • • • • • • • • • • • • • • •

ELLIOT MYERS, 73, hefts a concrete block to shoulder height. Balancing atop a shaky scaffold, he slaps mortar onto a garage wall. Then it's down to the ground again for another load of blocks. Tirelessly, he lifts and climbs under the hot summer sun.

Ask this white-haired, straight-backed farmer the secret of his vigor, and he'll shrug. While his wife, Mildred, sometimes cheerfully admonishes him to "act your age," Myers wouldn't dream of hanging up his dungarees. He's just too darned busy to be old.

Not long ago, Myers decided his steers and chickens could survive without him. He lit off for Australia and New Zealand on a month-long sojourn. Later, he trekked to Alaska to go one-on-one with salmon. Myers returned to his Pennsylvania homestead full of tales—and resolve to travel some more.

Myers is hale and hearty at an age when many are frail and ill. Today, there's no reason why Myers and others who've already passed the American male's average life span of 71 shouldn't enjoy many more years of full life.

NOTHING IS INEVITABLE

Gerontologists are finding ways to extend the period of productivity we associate with middle age into old age. As they make inroads into the mystifying continuum of birth to death, life extension—the big enchilada—seems within their reach. The outer limit anyone dares to speak about now is 120 years, but once the aging process is better understood, we may be able to shoot for 150 years.

The goal isn't simply a matter of finding ways for us to live longer, however. As writer Alexis Carrel once put it, "Longevity is only desirable if it increases the duration of youth, and not that of old age."

John W. Rowe, M.D., president of the Mount Sinai Medical Center in New York City, says gerontology's look into longevity is not so much at life span as at what he calls "health span."

That's what should concern you, too. Who needs to make it into the *Guinness Book of World Records* as the world's oldest man if that means enduring decades of pain and helplessness? But there will be plenty of takers for the prospect of middle age that stretches into the eighties.

There are a number of theories about why and how we age, each with its proponents and its critics. Some of the key theories suggest practical ways we can extend our health span and perhaps, ultimately, our life span.

A man born today can expect to live to 71. Life expectancy figures are averages, however, and not hard to beat. Roy Walford, M.D., 64, professor of pathology at the UCLA School of Medicine, thinks he's on to something that stacks the odds in your favor: "Nutrition above all else," he says.

Animal studies show a high-nutrient, low-calorie diet both

lengthens life and helps maintain a youthful demeanor. Dr. Walford calls the diet "undernutrition without malnutrition."

In simple terms, this means cramming as much good food as you can into 1,500 to 1,700 calories, about one-third fewer than the amount normally recommended for ideal weight and about one-half what most men now take in. Over several years, the diet will establish a new weight for you that will be 10 to 25 percent lower than when you began. Men on this diet should:

■ Avoid high-fat foods such as cheese, whole milk, and butter.

■ Eat low-fat proteins, especially fish and, if you must, very lean red meat.

■ Cut salt intake.

■ Drop sugary, fatty desserts.

■ Choose raw, unprocessed, natural foods, especially fruits and vegetables.

■ Aim to meet the government's recommended daily allowance (USRDA) of each nutrient within your caloric limit each day.

"It's really not difficult to eat this way," says Dr. Walford, who does just that. "You *can* change from your present diet, which is simply programming. When I was in central Africa, natives thought a meal wasn't complete unless one had a roasted palm grub. That's programming, too."

Dr. Walford claims that his diet is the only one he's found that consistently extended the life span of mice by 50 percent. Other attempts—with vitamin supplementation, exercise, drugs, oxygen therapy, surgery, and controlled temperature—came up short, merely maintaining the normal 40-month life of mice. "Calorie restriction, though, extends that span to 50-plus months," says Dr. Walford, who's written about his research in *The 120-Year Diet.*

Dr. Walford's colleague Richard Weindruch, Ph.D., points out that calorie-restricted mice not only live longer but remain physically and mentally vigorous longer than normal mice. When the scientists put food-restricted mice into mazes, they consistently out-learned mice on normal diets. "What's significant, too," he adds, "is that calorie restriction helps not only healthy mice but also disease-prone mice to live longer."

So far, diet restriction hasn't been tested scientifically in humans, but primate studies are planned. "Nutrition appears to play a major role in guarding against coronary heart disease, cancer, stroke, and other problems," says Dr. Weindruch, "and it may well turn out to be the key to slowing the aging process."

WHY AGE?

Denham Harman, M.D., Ph.D., professor of medicine and biochemistry at the University of Nebraska College of Medicine, first proposed another key theory of aging 30 years ago. Called the free-radical theory of aging, it is now considered by many researchers to be one of the most plausible explanations of why we get old and ill. It also offers hope that we can slow the course of aging by modifying our lifestyle.

Free radicals are created as unavoidable by-products of human metabolism. They are involved in important chemical reactions, such as breaking down foods to extract energy. Too many free radicals can gradually disrupt our most vital life processes, however. In fact, excess free radicals can begin to shut down the very mechanisms they were designed to serve.

How exactly do free radicals do their damage? It all starts with breathing: The oxygen we inhale reacts with compounds in the body to make energy. This oxidation process doesn't always go smoothly, however. "Fragments of molecules are frequently created that have an unpaired electron, and these are what we call free radicals," explains Dr. Harman. "They can be highly disruptive to other molecules they meet."

Scientists have already come up with at least 60 diseases associated with free radicals, among them heart disease, cancer, arthritis, Alzheimer's disease, and cataracts. In fact, the immune system itself may be vulnerable to free-radical attack, says Dr. Harman. Even some of Father Time's less welcome cosmetic adjustments—facial wrinkles and sagging jowls, for example—could be due to free radicals, which gradually erode the collagen that keeps skin elastic.

Stress seems to play a role in free-radical formation. "Stress . . . gives rise to free radicals, so any activity that combats stress is also going to combat free radicals," says Dr. Harman.

Activities other than smoking and drinking, that is. Tobacco and alcohol are two of the more prolific free-radical generators around. "A single puff of a cigarette results in the creation of over 1,017 free radicals," says William A. Pryor, Ph.D., of the Biodynamics Institute at Louisiana State University. This is also one of the reasons that cigarette smoking is such a potent cause of lung cancer. (See "Arresting Free Radicals" below for other contributors and protectors.)

Fortunately, our body has mechanisms for keeping these potential troublemakers in check. For example, vitamins A, C, and E and the trace element selenium are antioxidants, says Dr. Harman. Our bodies use these nutrients not only to reduce the damage created by free radicals but also to prevent their formation.

• •

ARRESTING FREE RADICALS

New research indicates that ill health and premature aging may result from proliferation within the body of free radicals—highly reactive molecules produced in response to environmental toxins and normal cellular metabolism. Here's how to keep the troublemakers in check.

Produce fewer by avoiding:

- Cigarette smoke
- Immoderate consumption of alcohol
- Intense sunlight
- X-rays
- Ozone
- Radon
- Pesticides
- Asbestos
- Cured meats
- Dietary fats in the blood
- Psychological stress
- Prolonged, exhaustive exercise
- Excess body fat

Neutralize more with:

- Vitamin A (carrots, cantaloupe, sweet potatoes)
- Vitamin C (citrus fruits, green peppers, cantaloupe)
- Vitamin E (wheat germ, nuts, peanut butter)
- Selenium (fish, Brazil nuts, rice)
- Stress reduction
- HDL cholesterol (encouraged by moderate daily exercise, weight loss, and a high-fiber, low-fat diet)
- Moderate daily exercise (gardening, walking, bicycling)

• •

Antioxidants appear to do this through a unique ability to scavenge unpaired electrons and render them harmless.

Experts disagree about the value of vitamin supplements, but they don't dispute the wisdom of getting adequate amounts of vitamins A and C in the diet naturally. Because vitamin E can be relatively difficult to get naturally, Dr. Harman recommends a supplement of about 200 international units (IUs) daily.

Free-radical activity is also promoted by low-density lipoproteins (LDLs), a form of cholesterol. Since exercise tends to boost high-density lipoproteins (HDL cholesterol), which drive down the level of LDLs, controlling weight through moderate exercise makes doubly good sense.

But you needn't knock yourself out. Studies suggest that moderate exercise, such as gardening and walking, may even be better than more strenuous activity. The reason? Mild exertion produces fewer free radicals than strenuous exercise and burns calories with less oxygen intake. And remember that cellular interaction with oxygen is one of the major sources of free-radical production in the first place. In fact, some research suggests that extreme and prolonged exertion may create free radicals to an unhealthful degree.

SLOWING THE HANDS OF TIME

So let's say you've cleaned up your junk food-filled, sedentary act. You're shooting for the century mark.

It's far from an impossible dream. By 1985, more than 25,000 people had hit that milestone, two-thirds more than just five years earlier. According to the *Statistical Bulletin,* more than 400,000 Americans will live to be 100 years old by 2025, a mere 33 years from now. By 2020, the number of Americans over a more reasonable age 85 will nearly double, to about 5 million people.

This neat trick has little to do with any genetic or biological improvements in the basic human machine, however. The stripped-down Neanderthal model might have survived just as long if he'd had the advantages of the late 20th century. Some scientists are now trying to tinker with such basic biological mechanisms as our genes in the hope of learning how to extend the human life span.

"The idea is futuristic, but it's not beyond the realistic imagination that once the mechanism of the aging process is known, it would be possible to change the process through bioengineering or some other technology so we could live longer," says Vincent J. Cristofalo, Ph.D., a cell biologist and director of the Center for the Study of Aging at the University of Pennsylvania. "I'm not saying it's going to happen soon, but it's no longer a crazy idea."

Bioengineering is among the most promising of the research techniques. Right now, geneticists are fascinated by a species of nematode, a type of worm, called *C. elegans*. Thomas E. Johnson, Ph.D., associate professor of behavioral genetics at the University of Colorado, Boulder, has bred nematodes that can live for five weeks, roughly 70 percent longer than normal. The secret of their longevity lies in a single gene, thought to be one of those responsible for aging in the worms. Among normal nematodes, this gene seems to number their days. But in the long-lived variety, the gene—appropriately christened *age-1*—has been altered by chemical mutation. The result: an older, though not necessarily wiser, mutant worm.

• •

Health Club 2000

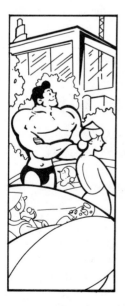

What do future health clubs have in store? According to Bob Goldman, D.O., founder and director of the National Academy of Sports Medicine, you could very well insert your computer card and the exercise machines call you by name, select the right amount of weight and number of reps at each resistance level, and tell you when you've reached your goal. After you're finished, the computer will print your progress report and recommend a program for you to follow next time. "Personalization will be the key to exercise equipment of the future," says Dr. Goldman. "The machines will adjust to the user's biomechanics: leg length, range of motion, and strength curve of body parts."

Dr. Johnson is quick to point out that this idea is still a long way from application in humans. Nematodes have roughly 5,000 genes; we have about 100,000. Man is a far more complex animal, and most of his genes aren't so well understood. Still, if there is a genetic basis for long life in this simple creature, the implications for humans are clear. If we could live 70 percent longer, 130-year-old men would be commonplace.

For now, though, we'll have to set our sights a bit lower. "The first wave will not be living to be 150," says Dr. Cristofalo. "It will be living to be 90, staying productive to the end."

In the absence of disease, the organs of an 80-year-old man function nearly as well as those of a 20-year-old. The heart, lungs, digestive system, and, most important, brain all adapt to old age in ways that have been measured in the laboratory. But efficiency is maintained only with effort. That means a good diet, regular exercise—and commitment.

Even those who've lived hard and fast (smokers, drinkers, hard-driving Type A personalities) can slow the hands of time if they start *right now*. "There is no point of no return," says Dr. Walford. "Whenever you start living right, you slow the rate of aging from that time on."

—*Connie Nesteruk*

The Appearance of Youth

Some hair and skin care advances offer hope, others, just hype. Can you tell them apart?

● ● ● ● ● ● ● ● ● ● ● ● ● ● ● ● ● ● ● ●

PROBABLY NO SIGNS of aging bother a man more than the ones that show above the shirt collar. Wrinkles, bags under the eyes, a hairline that's heading north—all visible signs to himself and others that the years are sneaking by. And forget what you've heard about The New Male Vanity; this stuff has been bugging men for centuries. In 4000 B.C., Egyptian men were rubbing ground animal parts on their heads in attempt to grow hair. That dumb wreath that Caesar wore was an early attempt at a toupee. John D. Rockefeller reportedly had a supply of fresh mother's milk delivered daily in the belief that it would keep his skin immune to aging.

The fact that, in the past, none of the miracle cures has ever proven to be more than snake oil has left many men resigned to a life of wearing hats and avoiding mirrors. Ironically, science is just now beginning to deliver on some of those broken promises. Researchers have been chipping away at the problems of wrinkling skin and disappearing hair for decades, and finally, there are some strategies, and even medicines, that offer an alternative to growing old ungracefully.

THE HAIR FACTS

First, let's look at what's happening on the front lines of hair restoration. Most men who lose their hair do so because they are genetically programmed to. Male pattern baldness is a trait that can be inherited from both parents. How it's passed on seems almost random. In many families, one son goes bald and the other does not.

If a man has a genetic predisposition to baldness, the rate of hair loss depends on his age and male sex hormones. Ten percent of men show obvious hair loss in their teens, 20 percent in their twenties, 30 percent in their thirties, and so on. Men who become substantially bald usually show significant hair loss by age 35.

Right now, the best treatment for male pattern baldness is the drug minoxidil, sold in the United States under the brand name Rogaine. After a long period of Food and Drug Administration (FDA) scrunity, minoxidil was approved as the first medical treatment for baldness. It appears to work by opening blood vessels in the scalp which had been too constricted for hair to grow.

In all the hype and hoopla over the discovery and approval of the drug, however, some men may have gotten the impression that it can work miracles. In most cases, it can't.

"The truth about this drug is that it will turn out to be great for some men but a huge disappointment for others," says Harry L. Roth, M.D., a clinical professor of dermatology at the University of California at San Francisco. Dr. Roth directed one of the 27 different year-long studies (involving 2,300 men) that were responsible for earning minoxidil its government approval. "It's important that men be forewarned of what minoxidil can and can't do, and for whom," Dr. Roth says. "Men who are older than 35 and whose baldness is quite extensive will not do well. The drug is most effective for men in their early twenties and thirties whose hair loss has started only within the past several years and is not advanced."

Elise Olsen, M.D., an assistant professor of medicine at the Duke University Medical Center who also directed an FDA minoxidil trial, agrees with Dr. Roth. "Men who have bald areas on the tops of their heads measuring 2 inches in diameter or less are the ones who will do best with this drug," Dr. Olsen says. "I would be reluctant to prescribe it for men whose conditions are considerably more advanced than that, unless of course their goal would be just to slow down their hair loss."

And indeed, even though minoxidil may not turn out to be the great baldness buster hoped for when this blood pressure drug's hair-raising powers were accidentally discovered 15 years ago, the stuff stands a good chance of at least being called a hair saver, which is certainly no small claim in its own right. "This could very well turn out to be minoxidil's greatest contribution," Dr. Roth says. "The FDA's studies did not examine this feature of minoxidil specifically, but the effect was widely observed. Even in men who saw no actual growth from minoxidil, most said they felt it at least slowed down their hair loss."

Other experts agree with the better-for-slowing-than-growing assessment. "The drug is clearly better for retarding hair loss than for growing new hair," says Gene T. Izuno, M.D., dermatologist at the Scripps Clinic in La Jolla, California, where another of the FDA's minoxidil trials was conducted. And according to Dominic Brandy, M.D., medical director of the Cosmetic Hair Replacement Surgery Center in Pittsburgh, "I will be prescribing minoxidil more as a defense against baldness than as a cure for it."

But of course, even already bald men will be coming to minoxidil with hope. Here are the facts they should be aware of when they do:

■ Minoxidil works best on men younger than 30 whose hair loss is not extensive and has started only recently, preferably within the last five years. Even among these prime candidates, only one-third can expect good results (at least a doubling in hair density), while about 40 percent can expect fair results (hair thickness doubling and a bald spot that will shrink but not disappear). The others will experience virtually no change, though they may experience a retarding of hair loss.

■ Minoxidil cannot grow new hair where there is none. It can only thicken and lengthen existing hairs.

■ Minoxidil won't do anything for a receding hairline; it cannot grow hair at the temples or forehead. It works best on bald spots on the top of the head measuring 2 inches in diameter or less.

■ Minoxidil must be applied twice daily for at least four to six months, and sometimes for a full year, before results are seen. At present, a year's supply costs about $700.

■ Minoxidil requires a lifetime commitment. A man who stops using it will lose whatever hair he has gained within about six months.

One thing is for sure: Minoxidil will not be the last word in medical treatments for baldness. The potential earnings from a real cure are mind-boggling, and every pharmaceutical company would love a piece. Research continues at a strong pace. (See "Beyond Minoxidil" on page 12.)

If you simply can't wait for science to get around to a dramatic cure, there are alternatives. "If a man is truly committed to having a significantly fuller head of hair, he can have it," says Dr. Brandy. Here's a quick rundown of procedures currently available.

The hair lift. Most recent and dramatic of the surgical alternatives is the hair "lift." In a series of three or four operations, bald scalp is removed, and scalp with hair is moved from the back and sides of the head to the top of the head. Results can be truly remarkable. Depending on how many operations are needed, costs range from $3,000 to $15,000.

Scalp reduction. Scalp reduction removes a section of bald scalp from the top of the head as the sides are drawn upward to minimize the size of the bald area. It's used when the bald spot is not large enough to warrant a full hair lift. Several operations can be performed a few months apart, the result being a reduction in the bald area. Prices for the procedure range from $500 to $2,000 per operation.

Hair transplants. The procedure, which has been around for over 30 years, takes plugs of hair from the back and sides of the head and surgically embeds them where hair is lacking. Plugs can vary in size from fairly large (8 to 20 hairs) to very small, some consisting of a single hair. Bad hair transplants are a very common problem, according to Dr. Brandy. "I've seen hundreds of bad trans–

plants in consultation, and I do a lot of repair work. A thorough job requires three or four operations. Otherwise, what you end up with looks like corn rows or picket fences." Prices range from $10 to $40 a plug, with a complete job costing about $6,000, depending on how many plugs are required.

Hair weaving. The procedure is not surgical but merely cosmetic in that it attaches extensions, either natural or synthetic, to existing hairs. On the downside, the extensions must be repositioned every four to six weeks as the hair grows out.

Hairpieces. Toupees seem to be out of favor with baby boomers. Hairpieces have gotten a bad name because so many men wear cheap ones that make them look as if a weasel died on top of their head. It's very hard to spot a good toupee, but the dreadful ones get noticed.

If you're thinking about a hairpiece, your best bet is to go to someone who makes a free consultation. Your best option is a cus-

• •

BEYOND MINOXIDIL

Minoxidil is the first medical treatment for baldness, but it won't be the last. A number of medications are currently under investigation. All of the drugs are *biologic response modifiers,* which means that, like minoxidil, they affect the basic control mechanisms of hair follicle development. None of the new agents can cause growth of new hair from follicles that have become defunct, however. All, like minoxidil, require a living hair follicle capable of stimulation. Here's a quick rundown of the drugs presently receiving the most attention. None has yet received FDA approval.

Viprostol. An antihypertensive agent whose effects thus far appear to be similar to, though slightly less dramatic than, minoxidil's.

Diazoxide. A potent antihypertensive and blood vessel dilator that some research has shown to be twice as effective as minoxidil.

Minoxidil plus Retin-A. A mixture that some studies suggest works better than minoxidil alone. The most important factor regarding minoxidil's efficacy seems to be how well it penetrates the scalp, and retinoic acid may improve that penetration, says Edward Bondi, M.D., of the University of Pennsylvania. Retin-A may also have some hair-stimulating properties by itself, according to some researchers.

• •

tom piece rather than an off-the-rack toupee. Synthetic pieces are better for active, sports-minded men because they hold up to weather and water better and are easier to keep clean. Natural pieces do tend to look slightly better at first, but the harsh processing done to Oriental hair—the largest hair source—makes the hair break down sooner. As for comparative costs, figure about $150 more for a natural piece than a synthetic piece in the $1,000 category.

SURFACE APPEARANCE

When it comes to their skin, men have an advantage over women. A man's skin is thicker, so it's less likely to wrinkle. But we're hardly immune. For the better part of three decades, our skin seems ageless. Then, slowly but surely—more slowly in some men than in others—tiny changes occur. The skin begins to lose its immunity to outside irritants. Sweat glands shrink, oil glands become less active, and we lose the benefit of their moisturizing capabilities. Wrinkles begin to form. They start where the skin is thinnest— around the eyes. Later, deeper wrinkles appear on the forehead and cheeks.

The degree to which you wrinkle is partly a matter of genetics. But only a small part of it is inevitable. In many cases, the skin breaks down because of photoaging—damage caused by too much exposure to the sun. The effect of this damage over a period of years

• •

A Not-So-Silly 18 Years Younger

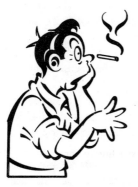

Nonsmokers outlive smokers by more years than previously thought, suggests a new study. Smokers at age 30 will live only to 65, on average, if they continue smoking, while 30-year-olds who have never smoked average 83— an 18-year difference. Earlier estimates of the gap ranged from 7 to 12 years, but that's because former smokers were grouped with lifelong nonsmokers, researchers say.

is what many people think of as aged skin—blotchy, lined, and leathery, with reduced elasticity. One of the most dramatic examples of sun damage I've ever seen was illustrated on a segment of the television show "20/20" last year. Co-host Hugh Downs showed pictures of an Indian woman who had spent most of her life outdoors side by side with those of a Tibetan monk who'd lived indoors for decades. She looked about 92 and he looked about 64. But he was 92 and she was 64.

"You don't have to be sunning for your skin to suffer the photoaging effects of the sun's ultraviolet rays," says Lorraine Kligman, Ph.D., assistant research professor in the Department of Dermatology at the University of Pennsylvania School of Medicine. "Photoaging occurs even when you're walking around doing your normal activities."

The answer isn't to become a monk, though. "Evidence suggests that if you start protecting your skin daily with a broad-spectrum sunscreen, skin that is already damaged will begin to repair itself," says Dr. Kligman. "Much of this repair work won't be visible for a long time. What you will see, however, is that your skin's blotchiness may tend to fade."

Dr. Kligman recommends that you wear a sunscreen with a sun protection factor (SPF) of 15 at all times. An SPF of 15 means that 15 hours in the sun will only add up to the damage that would occur in 1 hour if you were unprotected.

When you're on a fishing trip or doing anything else that keeps you out in intense sunlight for several hours, keep your nose and cheeks covered with zinc oxide cream, which will block nearly all the sun's rays.

Next to the sun, nothing will make you look old before your time quicker than smoking cigarettes will. Any experienced dermatologist will tell you he can spot a smoker at 10 yards by his "smoker's face"—heavy wrinkles around the eyes and mouth, poor skin tone, and gray pallor. Many doctors say they can see skin damage from smoking in men younger than 30.

Nicotine decreases blood flow to the skin by constricting vessels, and it inhibits the flow of nutrients to the cells of the skin. Tobacco also uses up vitamin C, a nutrient that's crucial to a healthy skin.

Beyond good care, there's always plastic surgery. More men are going under the knife than ever before, although surgery should probably be a last resort. A good face-lift can cost $10,000 and can require you to miss several weeks of work. For information on plastic surgery, call the Facial Plastic Surgery Information Service at (800) 332-3223.

—Paul Neimark

Staying Strong

With the right kind of upkeep, your body can be as tough at 50 as it was at 20—maybe tougher. The secret is training smart.

• • • • • • • • • • • • • • • • • • • •

JUST BECAUSE YOU don't find many over-40 men in those swinging-singles health clubs doesn't mean that older guys can't cut the mustard. I see men in their fifties, sixties, and even seventies working out all the time, but I usually find them at a body-building gym—the kinds of places with nothing but free weights and musty old leg machines. They're not there to socialize and pose in designer sweats; they're there to work hard and get strong. They know something that's escaped far too many middle-aged Americans: The older you get, the more beneficial strength training is for you.

It's no secret that cardiovascular improvement through aerobic exercise is a life extender and disease preventer. Armed with that knowledge, hordes of older Americans have hit the pavements with walking programs or have put in their time on stationary cycles. They're all the healthier for it.

But what about muscles? Once men hit middle age, they tend to shy away from strength training, even though there's no reason in the world *not* to do it and every reason in the world to do it. Older men stand to gain all the benefits from a stronger physique that younger men do: better overall health, improved posture, more power and stamina, a more attractive (and, it might be added, a younger-looking) body, and, perhaps most important of all, a bolstered self-image that translates into a bright, springy confidence.

"Strength training does add years to your life," says Frederick C. Hatfield, Ph.D., an exercise physiologist who runs the Consortium for Rehabilitation and Fitness Therapy Center in Reseda, California. "It's been proven again and again in recent years. But the main reason that people in their forties and fifties should train isn't for the *length* of their life but for the *quality* of their life. It's one thing to live to be 90 years old, but if you're feeble and helpless, you're not going to enjoy those years. Strength training beats aging by making life more worth living for longer."

Muscles are as able to respond to training in the fifth and sixth decades of life as they are in the third and fourth. Aging doesn't cause significant muscle cell loss. So since the object of weight training is to increase the size of muscle cells, not the number, you have virtually as much to work with at age 50 as you did at 25.

LIFTING INTO THE NINETIES

A Tufts University study of nursing-home residents who used weight training found that the elderly people were able to increase

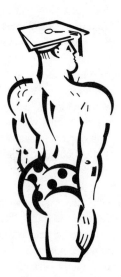

Pump Up Your Mind

If you think Hulk Hogan is dumb now, you should have seen him before he took up weight training. Scientists are discovering that exercise not only builds muscles but also may strengthen the brain. A neuropsychologist at the University of Illinois found that after four weeks of aerobic exercise, rats averaged a 20 percent increase in the number of blood vessels nourishing the cerebellum. He noted that improving the brain's ability to respond more efficiently to one form of exercise prepares it to better handle other types of physical activity—in rats and, we presume, in professional wrestlers as well.

their strength by as much as 200 percent and their muscle size by up to 15 percent. Even people in their nineties became stronger and increased the size of their muscles after working out on a Universal weight-training machine.

"You see lots of champion-caliber powerlifters who are stronger in their forties and even fifties than ever," says Dr. Hatfield, who counts himself among that group. Dr. Hatfield, now 46, set the world squat record at 1,014 pounds just a couple of years ago, and he's still competing.

So if building your muscles in your postyouth years helps you beat back the bugaboo of aging, why do so many older men avoid it? The reason probably has to do with the prevailing myth that as you get older, you necessarily get weaker. That's patently untrue, at least up until the age of 60. The fact is that there's less deterioration of muscles than other components of your body as time goes on. The medical community will tell you that until age 60, you'll probably retain 90 percent of your maximum strength—if you use your muscles. "There is some loss of elasticity," says Dr. Hatfield, "so what happens is people get lulled into believing that because they're feeling some changes with age, they can no longer train. That just isn't true. It's disuse, not use, that makes you lose strength in later years."

Actually, Dr. Hatfield contends, those men who have trained throughout their life might find that their workouts can be more and more beneficial as they get older. That's because muscle building is a complex endeavor, and your body responds in myriad ways, some more effective than others. Those in their forties and fifties have learned, perhaps subconsciously, the techniques and approaches that work best for them. They can do it better because they can do it smarter. "It's like rubbing sandpaper on your hand," says Dr. Hatfield. "Do it one way and you'll get calluses. Do it another and you'll get blisters. Do it regularly for 30 years and you know how to avoid the blisters and get calluses."

THE SOONER, THE BETTER

Of course, not everybody pushing 40 has been working out regularly throughout life, and many are concerned that budding middle age is not a safe time to start. Any responsible training advisor would recommend that men over 35 check with their doctor before starting up a weight-training program. It is true that the risk of

• •

SETTING THE PACE AT 75

Jerry Wible may be slowing down a bit. Twenty years ago, when he was 55, he could do a standing broad jump of 7 feet 3 inches. At last year's California Senior Olympics, his best jump was 6 feet 6 inches. Wible isn't letting this get him down, though. After all, he can still run a mile in under 7 minutes, and he won three medals at the North American Masters Track and Field Championships.

At 5 feet 10 inches and 165 pounds, Wible is in great shape for a man of 75 (or a man of 35). He's up at 5:30 every morning for 10 miles of running and walking. If there's a local track meet with a master's category, he'll enter that, or he'll spend some time training for the Senior Olympics. If the 10 acres of lawn at his Pennsylvania house need cutting, he does the job with a 21-inch push mower, the kind that runs on human power. When he travels, he always takes his running shoes. "I've run in 100 countries and on every continent," he says.

In addition to exercising daily, Wible watches his diet carefully. "I drink 2 or 3 quarts of water a day. No sodas. And I rarely drink alcohol. Not too much red meat and lots of fish. My cholesterol is 152. My resting pulse is 48 to 50."

His doctor is convinced Wible will live to be 100. Wible himself thinks he can do better. "Different articles claim we should be able to live to 125 or 140. Most people just don't take care of themselves."

—Ricki Stein

• •

injury or complications is greater after that age if you train incorrectly. The solution is simple: Train correctly.

"You can't shoot a cannon out of a canoe" is one of Dr. Hatfield's favorite expressions, one he uses with clients such as New York Met Sid Fernandez and sculpted pro football linemen Pete Koch and the recently retired Mark Gastineau. "You have to build a solid foundation. That's especially true with older trainees, who often want to concentrate on one body part, perhaps thinking they don't have the time for a well-rounded development. That's dangerous.

"For example, even at a very advanced age, you can learn to bench-press 300 pounds. But as you build up just your pectoral muscles to do that, you could blow out your shoulders or arms in the process. Older people especially must start very slowly with a total-body development program, and then work up gradually."

So does strength training "beat" aging? That is almost as much a philosophical question as a medical one. The modern medical community is nearly unanimous in the belief that regular vigorous exercise combats the kinds of diseases that older Americans are prone to, notably heart disease. Muscleheads like Dr. Hatfield are convinced that weight training adds years—and, of course, better quality—to your life. But nothing stops the clock.

What weight training really does is allow you to make a statement about what your life is going to be like as time passes. Most age-related sacrifices are the result of acquiescing to false notions of what you can or can't do as you get older; the best example of this is allowing your muscles to weaken because of the myth that there's nothing you can do about it.

Everybody has his own physical potential at any age, and the closer you get to it, the better your life will be. If you're 48 and you're hesitant about strength training because "in two years I'll be 50, for heaven's sake," you're cheating yourself. In two years, you're going to be 50 no matter what. It's a question of what kind of 50 you want to be.

—Kelly Garret

Age-Proof Your Mind

It's not how many brain cells you have, it's how much you continue to use them. Experts outline the very best mental exercises for staying sharp.

• •

ALL TOO OFTEN, older people *assume* that gears are slipping upstairs simply because they've had a certain number of birthdays. They fall prey to the myth that aging automatically brings with it a gradual breakdown in mental ability.

These assumptions had gone largely unchallenged until a few years ago, when research on aging brought about a new appreciation for the mind's resilience throughout life. Consider the following findings:

■ Although a modest impairment of some memory functions is a normal part of aging, most of us can expect to enjoy our good memories well into old age. Memory declines both are smaller and occur later in life than previously believed.

■ Brain cells *do* die in great numbers as we age. But we need far less than we have. Even at a clip of 50,000 to 100,000 neurons a day, we stand to lose only 1 billion of our 100 billion cells by age 70. Fortunately, the important variable here isn't the number of cells but the circuitry and chemistry that interconnect the billions and billions that do stay aboard.

■ Our mental abilities are tools that become sharper with use. You can't wear them out or use them up. As you grow older, you can consciously take on new challenges for the purpose of keeping your mind fit.

Science once held that the brain grows rapidly during early life and then, when we hit our twenties, settles down into a long slump. But research on aging has poked big holes in that scenario. The fact is, your brain is not fully developed at the end of your teens—or at 80, for that matter. Studies on laboratory animals suggest that your brain continues to grow as long as you continue to provide it with challenges and stimulation. The brain is a "plastic" organ, designed to increase its power to meet the demands we place upon it.

Of course, there are two sides to the story. What can be gained can also be lost. Your mental powers are vulnerable to an indifferent diet . . . they may wither through disuse, boredom, or a lack of self-confidence. "The brain, no less than the rest of the body, is subject to the 'use it or lose it' law," says Walter Bortz, M.D., former president of the American Geriatrics Society.

CARE AND MAINTENANCE

As the owner-operator of a brain, the responsibility is yours. Take care of the old gray stuff now, and it will try not to embarrass you later on. To that end, here's a sort of maintenance manual for your mind.

Exercise Your Mind

Memory, and a lot of other intellectual powers, can be strengthened. In *Stop Forgetting,* the late memory expert Bruno Furst made an analogy with building muscles: "If we realize that memory can be developed like a muscle, we must also accept the truth that its efficiency will diminish like a muscle if not properly used." Of course, staying mentally fit is as much a matter of retaining mental flexibility as of turning your memory into a steel trap for facts.

One of the best mental exercises for maintaining a fit, young mind is flexing your creativity. It's popularly accepted that we get less creative as we age, and some studies confirm that older people can be less flexible and creative thinkers. Apparently, something threatening to originality happens to many of us on the way to middle age. What could it be?

One study on the changing nature of creativity throughout life looked at ways in which younger and older subjects handled a creative writing assignment. The pieces were rated for creativity by three English professors based on criteria such as picturesqueness, vividness, original plot and setting, and humor. Generally, the younger subjects outperformed the older ones.

The study's findings suggest that older people tend to rely more on stored knowledge than on on-the-spot creativity. The researchers mention the demands of earning a living, keeping up a home, and raising children as possible reasons for the decline in creativity with advancing age. "None of this will set the stage for the time and concentration that the creative processes demand," concludes the study.

The researchers also point out that the ratings reflected each person's level of interest in the task. They suggest that older people can keep their creativity alive by cultivating their curiosity and enthusiasm about things throughout life.

It also appears that your mother was right: Television does rot your brain and deserves its nickname, "the boob tube." In one study, the number of hours spent watching TV was the best predictor of results on a creativity test and creative writing assignment—the more hours in front of the set, the lower the creativity ratings. Many of the lowest scorers even rated TV watching as their favorite activity. In contrast, the highest scorers said their favorite activity was spending time with friends.

Use Your Body to Enliven Your Brain

Researchers have found that physical exercise can keep your mind as fit and youthful as your body. The opposite is true as well. Physical inactivity seems to make the mind go flabby. It's known that a sedentary lifestyle is accompanied by electrical and chemical changes in the brain—a gradual winding down of brain-wave frequency and decreased levels of two neurotransmitters, dopamine and noradrenaline.

Marathoner George Sheehan, M.D., author of *Running and Being,* notes that lots of good things take place upstairs when he hits the road: "There is all the while a stream of consciousness, a torrent of ideas, coursing through my brain. One idea after another goes hurtling past like so much white water."

Writer John Jerome, who at age 47 decided to take up competitive masters swimming, has a similar outlook. As he explains in the book *Staying with It,* he began swimming laps to maintain the vitality of his nervous system, not simply to keep physically fit. He discovered during his hours in the pool that exercise can win back mental powers that had been diminished with disuse. As he put it: "If you ask a living organism for more, the organism will, within reason, respond. . . . To age, on the other hand, is to begin asking less." In other words, when a part of the body or mind is allowed to slow down, aging advances a step.

You don't have to be a competitive athlete to benefit your brain. Working out two or three times a week is enough, and apparently there's no real harm done by having back-to-back exercise days— good news for those who have to squeeze in their workouts on weekends. Research shows that the number of miles jogged or laps swum is not as important as simply getting out there regularly.

Eat Memorable Meals

A memory tonic has yet to hit the market. But one nutrient, choline, has been identified as a key to memory function. Ronald Mervis, Ph.D., director of Ohio State University's Brain Aging and Dementia Research Group, suspects that choline can help to retard the effects of normal aging on the brain, from midlife on. Choline has been credited with two major roles: It is the substance from which the brain makes acetylcholine, a neurotransmitter involved in memory function, and it may keep nerve cell membranes, including the synapses (the communication points between brain cells), intact.

Levels of acetylcholine characteristically drop as we age, particularly in people with Alzheimer's disease, the most common form of senility. But even for the great majority of older people who aren't troubled by senility, acetylcholine's effectiveness normally declines.

The reasons aren't known. Experts speculate, however, that the brain may be producing too little acetylcholine.

Choline has been used experimentally to slow memory loss in Alzheimer's patients, but young, healthy people are also affected by choline levels. One study showed that college students became forgetful, much as if they had aged prematurely, when acetylcholine levels were artificially lowered by a drug.

This is not to say that choline has been proven to have protective powers. But until its roles are well established, a choline-rich diet and a daily supplement over the years might be a safe and affordable form of nutritional insurance. A last-minute treatment with choline, on the other hand, is unlikely to bail out a person showing severe impairment, says Dr. Mervis.

Choline is present in many foods, mainly eggs, liver, peanuts, and soybeans, and in lecithin, a soybean product. Commonly used as an additive, lecithin improves the consistency of a variety of foods, including ice cream, mayonnaise, and margarine. The National Academy of Sciences says we typically get 400 to 900 milligrams of choline from our diet each day, but no Recommended Dietary Allowance (RDA) has been set.

Sheldon Saul Hendler, M.D., Ph.D., author of *The Complete Guide to Anti-Aging Nutrients,* cautions that if you want to take supplements, you should take no more than 1 gram of supplemental choline or 10 grams of lecithin per day. Larger doses can cause nausea, vomiting, and dizziness. (Of course, you shouldn't take this or any supplement without your doctor's approval and supervision.)

Go Easy on the Alcohol

Alcohol can be unfriendly to mental function at any age. Predictably, alcohol's mind-pickling effect is most pronounced in heavy drinkers. Chronic alcoholism may speed up the decline in mental performance that normally accompanies aging. As a cause of progressive dementia, alcoholism ranks fourth. That's chilling evidence for habitual drinkers. But what about the great majority of men who take their alcohol in moderate, occasional doses?

A summary of research on social drinking found that "moderate doses of alcohol impair . . . abstracting ability, information processing, and, in particular, memory." What's more, these abilities show deficits even when social drinkers are tested sober.

This news is tempered somewhat by evidence that the brain

can forgive as well as forget. Alcoholics who were tested four or five weeks after starting treatment for their addiction performed remarkably well on memory tests.

Not everyone is equally susceptible to alcohol's effects on the brain, according to Charles Golden, Ph.D., professor of neuropsychology at Drexel University. "It's not so much the amount of alcohol that matters, it's an individual's reaction to it," he says. People who seem to overreact to even small amounts of alcohol—who experience marked personality changes or blackouts or confusion—might consider themselves especially susceptible.

Relax

Stress can prematurely age your mind. Memory expert Arthur Bornstein has called heavy stress the number one enemy of a good memory. Here are some of the most effective ways to unwind.

Meditation. Meditation means many different things, ranging from taking a moment to collect thoughts to highly structured forms of Eastern meditation. One study in the *International Journal of Neuroscience* suggests that meditation may actually slow the aging process. People who practiced Transcendental Meditation (TM) were compared with nonmeditators on three biological indicators of aging: hearing, vision, and blood pressure. For each subject, a biological age was calculated and then contrasted with his or her actual, chronological age.

It turned out that long-term TM meditators had a biological age that averaged 12 years younger than their actual age; those who had been meditating a relatively short time averaged 5 years younger; and the controls, who did not meditate, averaged 2.2 years younger.

No one knows exactly how meditation works. Some studies have pointed to changes in the central nervous system; others, to improved mental efficiency that results from reducing the steady stream of mental chatter.

If you feel uncomfortable at the thought of relying on lotus positions and mantras, you might want to try a simple, Westernized form of meditation developed by cardiologist Herbert Benson, M.D. Far from anything mystical, his "relaxation response" technique draws on an intentionally mundane mantra—the syllable *one*. Twice a day, the meditator sits comfortably in a quiet place and repeats that syllable silently. That's it.

Dr. Benson says this easy practice can help mute the ravages of the fight-or-flight syndrome, the body's automatic way of preparing for danger through a release of adrenaline and noradrenaline. This is a healthy reaction, so long as the increased level of hormones translates to physical action. But if we just sit on our anger and fear and allow the emotional storm to brew within, all kinds of physiological thunder ensue: elevated blood pressure, pounding heart, tense muscles—all the wear and tear that ages our bodies and minds.

Biofeedback. A modern technological version of meditation is biofeedback. In fact, biofeedback can be thought of as "machine-assisted meditation," explains Ken Pelletier, Ph.D., a psychologist who specializes in stress management. Using an apparatus that monitors brain waves, muscle activity, or other bodily functions, a person can learn to control heart rate, blood pressure, and skin temperature, much as an Indian yogi does. When the subject manages to alter a biological state, such as muscle tightness, the machine provides the immediate "feedback" that the change has in fact taken place. This technique is used to treat problems such as high blood pressure, heart disease, gastrointestinal problems, and migraine headaches.

Beware of Drug Side Effects

A number of drugs can undermine mental functioning. Unfortunately, older people are most adversely affected by drugs—they take more kinds of drugs than younger people, and they can least afford the loss. Drugs that may impair memory include barbiturates and other sedatives, benzodiazepines, tricyclic antidepressants, antihistamines, certain anticonvulsants, diuretics, and tranquilizers—Valium in particular.

If you suspect a drug is affecting your mental faculties, ask your doctor, read the literature that came with the product, or go straight to the library and consult the *Physicians' Desk Reference*. Your doctor may cut the dosage, switch you to another drug, or discontinue it altogether.

WHAT'S ON THE HORIZON

The search for mental elixirs continues, and from time to time, hints of success are reported in medical journals and the popular press. While there's nothing out there now to get excited about, a couple of recent findings offer promise for future treatments.

Researchers in the Netherlands and at the National Institute of Mental Health reported that Vasopressin, a drug prescribed to encourage the kidneys to retain water, improved performance on memory tests by both college students and older people. So why hasn't Vasopressin become a household word? First, the drug can have dangerous side effects. However, one form of the drug is reported to restrict its power to the memory. Once this new, improved version undergoes testing, it may ultimately find its way into our medicine chests before we become too old to remember to take it.

Hydergine is a drug that has been prescribed to counteract the effects of aging on the brain and to revive the memory in particular. It may work by enhancing the effectiveness of certain neurotransmitters. Dr. Hendler calls the drug "a very promising substance that may eventually be shown to have a protective role against dementia." But he cautions that researchers still do not know enough about Hydergine's long-term effects or its value in preventing mental decline. While this drug is now available by prescription only, perhaps one day drugs like Hydergine and Vasopressin will be as ready a remedy for mental slippage as aspirin now is for a headache.

Mental stretching, physical exercise, proper diet, reducing stress—these are your bulwarks against mental decline. They can help you make the most of the brainpower you were born with—an important point, given that we have the same brain that served our prehistoric, club-wielding ancestors. The difference between them and us isn't mental wattage; it's the environment in which the brain develops. That's the real key to staying sharp, regardless of chronological age. And best of all, it's something you can control and use to your best advantage.

—Roger Yepsen

Aging Gracefully, Inside and Out

Here's one guy who's old enough to be playing Grandpa, but Hollywood (and most of America) still thinks he's sexy. Here's the verdict on Paul Newman.

• •

YOU CAN'T TALK ABOUT how men stay young without talking about Paul Newman, even if Paul Newman doesn't want to talk about it.

I mean, does this guy look like he was born in 1925? He's 13 years older than Redford, but he's got fewer wrinkles. He's 3 years older than George C. Scott, but Newman doesn't look nearly time-worn enough to pull off those presidential parts that Scott gets. In fact, he still gets to play romantic leads with women who are decades younger.

It's not just those lit-from-within blue eyes, either, although they certainly don't hurt his looks. If Newman were bald and jowly, the eyes might pull him through. But the point is, he's *not* bald or jowly, so the eyes are just a bonus.

My assignment was to find out how Newman does it. How has he managed to look and act so youthful at an age when many men begin to feel old? I figured Newman must have a lot of insight into this. Clearly he thinks about it, since men don't age this gracefully without some effort. I figured he and I would sit down for a chat and I'd pick his brain for a little advice the rest of us can use. We live in the same town (Westport, Connecticut), so it wouldn't be a problem to drive on over to his place—a Revolutionary War–era farmhouse on 11 acres—for a Budweiser and some chat. Maybe he'd even offer a bowl of his famous popcorn to help me work up a thirst.

A call to Newman's public relations people put a quick end to that notion. The word came back from Newman that he didn't want to talk. He said he's "tired of being portrayed as the perennially youthful man."

We should all have such problems. I can't actually recall anyone ever calling me a perennially youthful man, but if someone did, I guarantee I wouldn't get tired of it for a long time.

But okay, I can understand his feelings. Newman's reached an age where he wants to be appreciated for his work as a serious actor, not as a hunk of meat. He eschews vanity and the whole Hollywood thing. And after all, this is a guy who can't go out in public without some lady stopping him and saying, "Take off your sunglasses, I want to see your blue eyes." (These encounters, he has said, continue to annoy him, even after all these years: "It's like saying to a woman 'Open your blouse, I want to see your chest.' ") But public postures aside, the man *is* perennially youthful, even if he's tired of being reminded, and I suspected he works damned hard at it.

My approach to getting the story was going to have to change, though. Instead of getting it directly from the source, I was going to have to read everything about the man I could get my hands on, talk to his friends and business associates, and make a few educated guesses.

NO NEED FOR TOUCHED-UP PHOTOS

First, I wanted to establish that Newman's youthful looks weren't achieved by makeup, photo retouching, or some other movie magic. Nope, his friends say, he looks that good at the grocery store on Saturday morning, too. Every single one told me he doesn't look *nearly* his age. I heard descriptions like "reed-thin," "almost perfectly proportioned," "holds himself ramrod straight." His height may be debatable (5 feet 10 inches is the official word, although some wags in the tabloid world claim he's shorter), but the wise-guy half-smile and see-through-you blue eyes are incontrovertible. Sure, his family calls him Old Skinny Legs, the hair has gone silver, and little lines are starting to appear below his mouth, but according to Howard Pearson, M.D., medical director of Newman's Hole in the Wall Gang Camp and professor of pediatrics at Yale University School of Medicine, the actor is "lean, hasn't lost his hair, and has an excellent complexion."

Don Kulowski, president of Century Pools in New Britain, Connecticut, and the guy who installed the big pool at Newman's camp, views the actor with admiration and envy. "He's in excellent shape. He's slight, not overweight, and appears to have nonstop energy. He looks like he's in his forties. I'm ten years behind him, and I'd like to be in that kind of shape."

As for the reasons, heredity certainly played a starring role. Newman was the recipient of a good set of genes. If you saw those magazine ads his older brother, Arthur, did for an investment company, you know that youthful looks run in the family. Getting good genes is lucky. Excellent physical shape is work. Newman works. Buddy Dinan, the owner of Westport Pool and Spa, has installed two hot tubs and a spa for the Newmans. He says the Blue-Eyed One "swims laps, jogs a lot, and does a daily Danish plunge: from sauna to hot tub to cold tub." Dinan sees in Newman, besides a "friendly guy, great to deal with, not aloof," a man with a "strong commitment to life and staying healthy."

Besides the swimming, jogging, and saunas, Newman works out on an exercise bike and weight machines every day while watching cable news. Because he has a tendency toward a beer gut, he also does a lot of sit-ups on a slant board. A few years ago, he did so many he gave himself a hernia.

Peter Bush, a Connecticut disc jockey who's been involved in sports car–racing promotions with Newman, describes the actor as being in "exceptional condition for someone his age. He's a classic case of 'You think young, you are young.' He works out regularly, and he makes sure all his parts check out. He has the reaction time of someone much younger."

"He's physically fit," agrees Peter Slater, vice president of the Newman-Sharp Racing Team, adding that for what an endurance racer goes through, Newman had better be. According to Slater, it's fairly unusual for a man in his sixties to be this good, but Newman still has what it takes: dexterity, coordination, concentration, the ability to handle stress.

About the only aspect of Newman's health regimen with an aura of mystery about it is the ice. Life magazine says he "believes in the mysterious preservative powers of ice—in healing and in tightening skin"—and that he likes to dunk his face in a sink of ice cubes for a few seconds every morning. Nuh-uh, says the *New York Times Magazine:* Just a rumor.

AVOIDING DIETARY SINS

In keeping with the anti-star, regular-guy image that's so important to him, Newman—at least in public—is not a fussy eater. At the racetrack, he'll grab a convenience-store lunch of a ready-made sandwich and grape soda pop. While directing, he'll nosh on salty popcorn from a plastic garbage bag. And he's been known to stop by the Westport Häagen-Dazs occasionally for a vanilla ice cream bar with milk chocolate and peanuts, although perhaps less often since the time a fellow customer got so flustered at coming face-to-face with Newman's baby blues that she put her ice cream cone into her pocketbook before exiting.

Although none of the above qualifies as a dietary sin, Newman's real care and feeding habits are more in evidence in his private life. And *here* we see a man who cares about *food*. For years he gave a vinaigrette salad dressing of his own concoction to his best friends as Christmas gifts. Eventually he created Newman's Own, Inc., an all-natural line of foods with Newman's Own Salad Dressing as the headliner (supported by spaghetti sauce, popcorn, and lemonade). Newman is a man who as often as not dons the chef's toque in his own family (his daughter Nell calls him a "risk taker—with almost flawless results") and won't think twice about driving out for fresh ingredients for his specialties. A man who, with best buddy A. E. Hotchner, well-known writer and fellow Westporter, coauthored *Newman's Own Cookbook*.

Newman "eats lightly," according to Dr. Howard Pearson, who remembers a recent Newman meal of tiny clams on the half shell, angel hair pasta, and scrod with capers. The clam dish is a favorite Newman appetizer; he describes it with loving precision in his cookbook: "A dozen tiny clams on the half shell, topped with a squirt of lemon juice and a dollop of fresh horseradish—but *never* that dread spicy-catsup cocktail sauce! If baby clams are not available, I'll settle for a plate of celery hearts chopped fine in an oil-and-vinegar dressing, which I concoct." His favorite sandwich reportedly is sliced cucumbers on whole wheat.

Newman's only habit that could conceivably be considered a potential vice is the ubiquitous Bud. "If Budweiser went out of business," says Don Kulowski, "Newman would go out of business." On the other hand, Newman hasn't touched hard liquor for years, and there's some evidence that moderate drinking may actually be a healthy habit: A study from the Institute for Aerobics Research in Dallas, for example, has shown that moderate quantities of alcohol seem to lower the risk of heart disease; other studies show a tipple now and then can contribute to longer life. An occasional wine or beer also can mildly sedate the day's jitters and bolster emotional well-being—both important in staving off aging.

FEELING GOOD BY DOING GOOD

When you think about secrets of graceful aging, you think in terms of fitness, diet, genes—and "other." It's obvious that Newman does pretty well on the first three. Where he really hits the jackpot is in the "other." Newman's at a stage and status in life where he could easily sit back; instead, he's *giving* back. As in doing unto others. As in altruism. And doctors and researchers are now finding that people with an altruistic spirit tend to stay healthier and live longer. The converse of this seems to be true, too: According to research done by Larry Scherwitz, Ph.D., at the Medical Research Institute of San Francisco, self-centered people are much more likely to die of a heart attack than less self-centered people.

Altruism is the main ingredient in Newman's Own, Inc. Almost everyone knows that venture started as a goof; not everyone knows it's now a multimillion-dollar business that plows *all* its profits into charity. The American Foundation for AIDS Research, the Cystic Fibrosis Foundation, the American Ballet Theatre, the Central Park Conservancy, and the Scott Newman Foundation (named for his son, who reportedly died of an accidental overdose of alcohol and drugs) all have benefited from Newman's generosity.

The main beneficiary these days is Newman's Hole in the Wall Gang Camp, which opened last summer in Ashford, Connecticut. It's a summer camp for kids from 7 to 17 who have cancer or potentially fatal blood diseases. "The idea for the camp was just there, full-blown, one morning," Newman says. "I've had friends who died young. Life is whimsical. Longevity is an incredible gift, and some people don't get to enjoy it."

According to Dr. Howard Pearson, Newman's presence was nothing like "the general view we have of the celebrity who gives to philanthropic causes, the one who comes to the tux-and-black-tie kickoff and then runs out." Dr. Pearson says Newman "oversaw every aspect, from the site selection to the architectural design to the landscaping and the furnishings in the cabins. He took an intimate and continuing part. If there was a meeting with the septic-tank people, he'd be there!"

Don Kulowski marvels at the way Newman mobilized and motivated all the disparate contractors who pitched in at The Hole in the Wall Gang Camp: "He'd give each his undivided attention—for 90 seconds." Kulowski says Newman made a point of having a few beers with the guys on the construction crew and found a way to make everyone feel important. Peter Bush says it's involvement in causes like the camp that allows Newman to be at peace with himself: "His endless dedication to charitable causes makes him want to wake up every morning and look at the bright side."

FAMILY TIES

The image I like best is Newman as family man. His relationship with Joanne Woodward is by all accounts a solid one after more than 30 years of marriage. Newman has five daughters: Susan and Stephanie from his first marriage to actress Jackie Witte, and Nell, Melissa, and Clea with Woodward. Although he gives himself only one thumb-up as Dad, it's clear from the people around him that nothing means more to him than his family. Sometime co-star and young sidekick Tom Cruise wraps it nicely: "He lives a normal life. He's got several businesses, a wife, a family. That's good for me to see."

Loving family, devoted friends—another big longevity plus for Newman. Scientists are pretty confident that the more socially isolated a man is, the less healthy he is psychologically and physically, and the more likely he is to die. Conversely, they suggest, the better his social and family relationships, the longer he's likely to live.

Then there's Newman's sense of humor. Doctors say the ability to have a good laugh is very good for you. It's obvious from the Newman's Own product literature, and from just about every interview the actor has ever given, that he doesn't take himself very seriously. He's said to love a good prank and to be a willing audience for even the corniest joke. As Lindsay Crouse, an actress who worked with Newman on a couple of films, once told an interviewer: "After a serious scene, I'll say to him, 'Hey Paul, you hear the one about . . . ?' Then I tell him the last joke I heard, and no matter how bad it is, he's the best audience. The worst gag will break Paul up—he's on the *floor* laughing. There's a great willingness in him to play."

Finally, there's the racing. There's little doubt that the sport helps keep him young. "To be behind the wheel of a car doing over

100 mph is one of the most exhilarating things I know," he says. "Racing is a way of being a happy child again."

He also drives to test himself and to fight complacency. "You have to keep things off balance," he says, "or it's all over." Newman does little else besides race sports cars from April through October, and he's gotten very good at it—four times national champion in his class, and a billing by veteran driver Sam Posey as "one of the top endurance racers in the world."

According to Peter Slater of the Newman-Sharp Racing Team, Newman "has the mental outlook of a young, active person." Peter Bush says Newman "drives with the best of them. He's still got the fire. There's a lot of talk of his retiring from racing—but I know for a fact he'll be back next year."

TAKING THE YEARS IN STRIDE

So there it is. Paul Newman may be tired of his youthful image, but he seems to be doing all the right things to make sure it endures. He works out regularly and is careful about what he eats. He regularly tests himself and doesn't let boredom drag him down. He continues a love affair with his wife, and he has friends who are almost eerily devoted to him. And in what could be a crazy world of the rich and famous, he keeps things simple and sane: drives a Volkswagen Rabbit, does his own shopping, cooks his own food. As A. E. Hotchner told me, "He has a vital interest in life and surrounds himself with vital people."

Maybe the real secret behind Newman's graceful aging is his ambivalence about it. Beyond taking good care of himself, he refuses to be *obsessed* with aging gracefully. That's why he turns down interviews having to do with things like his appearance and takes on roles like Frank Galvin, the strung-out, over-the-hill lawyer in *The Verdict.* The primary factor in Newman being as young-acting as he is, says Don Kulowski, is that he doesn't dwell on his age.

—Hank Herman

Part 2

HEALTHY
EATS

Bat Away Fat

*The secret of a lean diet begins with what you throw
in your supermarket cart. The nutrition labels
often tell you all you need to know—but do you know
how to read them?*

••••••••••••••••••••••

THE BATTLE AGAINST a high-fat diet is won or lost in the supermarket. If your willpower or good sense fails you there, the fight is
lost. Because let's face it, once you bring home the bacon, it *owns*
you. If it gets into your refrigerator, it's going to get into you.

Make no mistake. This fight is a worthwhile one. Dietary fat is
a major risk factor for heart disease and some cancers. One study,

for example, suggests that by limiting fat to less than 25 percent of calories, we can stop new cholesterol buildup in the coronary arteries. Plus, fat is considered enemy number one in the battle of the bulge: Research shows that lean people get about 29 percent of their calories from fat; overweight people get about 35 percent.

A worthy goal to work toward is reducing the calories you get from fat to approximately 25 percent of your total caloric intake, a level many experts now feel is low enough to prevent problems in most men. This doesn't mean that every food you eat has to be one-quarter fat or less, but it does mean that 25 percent should be your overall average.

Things can get tricky at the market because many foods that are labeled "reduced fat" or "lower fat" may still be too high in fat. ("Reduced" simply means it has less fat in it than it used to. Maybe it used to have tons and now it only has a lot.) There are two easy ways you can protect yourself from misleading claims and lower the fat in your diet. Both involve reading the labels before you buy.

TRICKY LABELS

Most packaged foods carry a list of ingredients and nutrition information on their labels. However, they don't have to present that information in a way that's especially easy to understand.

• •

Sour Power

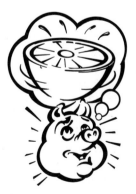

A two-year study of pigs has shown that adding one fresh grapefruit to the daily diet may help keep arteries clear of cholesterol plaque. "Based on this research, I would advise my patients with high cholesterol levels to eat a low-fat diet, get some exercise, and eat at least one grapefruit or several fresh oranges every day," comments James Cerda, M.D., one of the doctors who performed the study. And where does Dr. Cerda work? Why, the University of Florida's College of Medicine, of course.

The fat content of foods is almost always listed in grams—not a whole lot of help on the face of things. But by using a couple of simple rules of thumb, you can translate this into the information you need.

First, the Nine Rule: There are 9 calories in 1 gram of fat. So, to calculate the percentage of fat calories in any food, check the label for grams of fat and calories per serving, then plug into this formula: (grams of fat × 9 ÷ total calories) × 100 = percent of calories from fat.

For example: A bag of potato chips says each 160-calorie serving has 10 grams of fat, so you multiply those 10 grams by 9 (90), then divide by total calories (160), which gives you 0.56. Multiply by 100, and you'll find that those chips are roughly 56 percent fat.

Second, the Counting Rule: You can keep track of the fat in your diet simply by counting the grams. The average man takes in about 2,400 calories per day. If you're like him, you should be eating no more than 67 grams of fat per day. If you eat less, say 2,200 calories, you should eat no more than 61 grams of fat per day. If you eat more, 2,600 or 2,800 calories, for instance, your maximum fat intake should be 72 or 78 grams per day, respectively.

If you're not sure whether you fall into the category of an average eater, you can keep a log of your intake. Using one of those calorie-counter guides they sell at supermarket checkouts, note the number of calories in every food and beverage you consume over a few typical days. Then average the daily intakes together. Be careful, though. If the calorie guidebook lists calories for a 3-ounce portion of steak and your usual serving is 6 ounces, make sure you double the figure listed in the book.

Armed with that information, you can see that the 10 grams of fat in a single ounce of those chips is no small potatoes. Neither is the fast-food double cheeseburger that weighs in at a whopping 37 grams of fat nor the cup of premium ice cream at 34 grams of fat.

So whether you count percentages or grams, you should start counting. Your health, as well as your waistline, is depending on you. With that in mind, consider these strategies:

■ Don't shop on an empty stomach. Then your good sense will not have to be fighting bad advice from hungry taste buds.

■ Stick to your list. The people who design supermarkets are no fools. They position the "impulse items"—candy, Ding Dongs, cookies, and crackers—where they'll be sure to catch your eye. Unless the item is a decidedly healthful one, let it be.

■ Don't be afraid to experiment with new "reduced-fat" fare (just don't take their word for it; read that label). There are a number of satisfying, even downright tasty, low-fat cheeses, pastries, soups, and frozen foods out there. Don't make a judgment after the first bite. Your taste buds and pleasure centers need some time to adapt.

—Porter Shimer

The High-Nutrition Superstars

Here are 25 of the finest foods for fitness. Find your best sources of protein, vitamins, minerals, and fiber.

• • • • • • • • • • • • • • • • • • •

FOOD IS FUEL. It's simple, but it's true. Just as high-octane gas powers a car more efficiently, high-nutrient food delivers more energy to your body. If you want to be faster and stronger—if you want to last longer—you've got to use premium fuel.

Athletes have long tinkered with their diet to find the ideal foods for performance. And today, it's pretty widely agreed that a diet high in carbohydrates, modest in protein, and—most important—low in fat delivers the most nutritional value. Even if you're not an athlete, your food choices make a big difference in how you feel. Eating right means feeling more alert and creative at work, less prone to afternoon blahs. "A couch potato and a marathon runner should eat the same foods," says Nancy Clark, registered dietitian and director of nutrition services at Sportsmedicine Brookline.

But getting your diet right isn't as easy as pulling up to the pump and pushing the "super" button. Not all carbohydrate sources are created equal. Some pack a more powerful punch than others, delivering more vitamins and minerals at a lower calorie cost. Likewise, some protein sources are richer and leaner than others.

While no single "perfect food" exists, many stand out as nutritional superstars. Following, in alphabetical order, is a guide to the good stuff: 25 first-class foods.

BANANAS

The perfect portable snack. They're one of the richest sources of potassium, which may help regulate blood pressure, and a good source of fiber. Frozen banana chunks make a terrific guilt-free dessert. Bananas are also a natural antacid, according to a study published in the *Lancet*.

One banana has 105 calories, 0.5 gram of fat, 27 grams of carbohydrate, 1.2 grams of protein, 1 milligram of sodium, 0 milligrams of cholesterol, 2.2 grams of fiber, and 451 milligrams of potassium.

BEANS

An excellent source of fiber (important for keeping blood sugar and cholesterol levels under control). In fact, beans provide even more soluble fiber than oats. They're also high in protein and a good source of folate, a B vitamin important for building protein and red blood cells.

An average ½-cup serving has 112 calories, 0.4 gram of fat, 21 grams of carbohydrate, 7.5 grams of protein, 1 milligram of sodium, 0 milligrams of cholesterol, 7.7 grams of fiber, 304 milligrams of potassium, and 11 percent of the USRDA for folate.

BEEF

Lots of people have been beef bashing lately, but truly lean beef is a great source of zinc, high-quality protein, and iron. (The body absorbs the iron in meat more readily than the iron found in legumes, vegetables, or breads.) Still, you need to be picky about the meat that you buy. Choose only the leanest cuts, such as shank, round, flank, and chuck. Look for "select" grades and trim fatty edges before cooking. Supermarkets now routinely offer "¼-inch trim" cuts, with the fat trimmed super close. You may also be able to find a new type of cut: the "total trim," from which virtually all fat has been removed. These cuts are more expensive and are sold in smaller portions to help control serving sizes.

A 3-ounce serving of lean round steak has 163 calories, 5 grams of fat, 0 grams of carbohydrate, 27 grams of protein, 56 milligrams of sodium, 69 milligrams of cholesterol, 0 grams of fiber, 13 percent of the USRDA for iron, 32 percent of the USRDA for zinc, and 41 percent of the USRDA for vitamin B_{12}.

BROCCOLI

A wonder food—one of the best nutrition bets around. Not only is broccoli high in fiber and vitamin C, but it also provides folate, calcium, magnesium, and iron.

A 1-cup serving, cooked, has 46 calories, 0.4 gram of fat, 9 grams of carbohydrate, 5 grams of protein, 16 milligrams of sodium, 0 milligrams of cholesterol, 4.8 grams of fiber, 164 percent of the USRDA for vitamin C, 42 percent of the USRDA for vitamin A, 18 percent of the USRDA for calcium, and 24 percent of the USRDA for folate.

BROWN RICE

A good source of complex carbohydrates that provides twice as much fiber as white rice. Moreover, it beats white rice for almost every nutrient, including zinc, magnesium, protein, vitamin B_6, and selenium.

A ½-cup serving has 116 calories, 0.6 gram of fat, 25 grams of carbohydrate, 2.5 grams of protein, 0 milligrams of sodium, 0 milligrams of cholesterol, and 0.6 gram of fiber.

CARROT JUICE

Probably the most concentrated source of beta-carotene, which, in addition to its possible role as a cancer fighter, may play a key role in preventing the formation of cataracts later in life. Beta-carotene, a source of vitamin A, also may boost your immune system's ability to fight bacterial and viral infections, according to Joel Schwartz, Ph.D., associate professor at the Harvard School of Dental Medicine.

A ½-cup serving has 49 calories, 0.2 gram of fat, 11 grams of carbohydrate, 1 gram of protein, 36 milligrams of sodium, 0 milligrams of cholesterol, 1.2 grams of fiber, and about 33 percent of the USRDA for vitamin A.

CHICKEN

Three ounces of skinless chicken breast has only 3 grams of fat and contains vitamin B_6, a nutrient important for metabolizing protein. Dark meat has more fat than white but also more B vitamins, iron, zinc, and other nutrients. About skin: The usual advice is to cook the bird without it. (A thigh with skin can contain as much fat as beef.) But skin fat doesn't "migrate" into chicken meat, according to a letter in *The New England Journal of Medicine.* You may want to leave the skin on to keep the meat from drying out while cooking. Just don't give in to eating the crispy stuff later.

A 3-ounce breast with no skin, roasted, has 140 calories, 2.9 grams of fat, 0 grams of carbohydrate, 26 grams of protein, 62 milligrams of sodium, 0 grams of fiber, 58 percent of the USRDA for niacin, and 25 percent of the USRDA for vitamin B$_6$.

CORN

An often-overlooked source of fiber and carbohydrate. Sure, fresh corn tastes best, but frozen or canned alternatives are convenient ways to get additional fiber in your diet. Corn also has almost no fat.

A ½-cup serving has 67 calories, 0.6 gram of fat, 17 grams of carbohydrate, 2.5 grams of protein, 4 milligrams of sodium, 1.6 grams of fiber, and 17 micrograms of folate.

DRIED FRUIT

Because most of the water has been removed, dried fruits are terrific concentrated sources of energy and good sources of iron—a mineral that helps prevent anemia. High in fructose, they also can be intensely sweet, making them great desserts or snacks—and they're fat-free. The following data are for dried apricots; pears, figs, and raisins are similar.

A 3-ounce serving has 203 calories, 0.4 gram of fat, 53 grams of carbohydrate, 3.1 grams of protein, 8.5 milligrams of sodium, 0 milligrams of cholesterol, 6.8 grams of fiber, 22 percent of the USRDA for iron, and 123 percent of the USRDA for vitamin A.

FAT-FREE YOGURT

Among the few truly excellent sources of calcium—452 milligrams per 8-ounce carton—and riboflavin, yogurt's also a strong source of vitamin B$_{12}$. Use it to reduce fat in your diet: Substitute it for sour cream in casseroles or sauces; mix with herbs for vegetable dip; blend with fruit for a thick drink; stir into soups to make them creamy. Frozen, it's an excellent substitute for ice cream. To cut calories in half in flavored yogurts, choose brands artificially sweetened with aspartame (NutraSweet).

An 8-ounce serving (plain) has 127 calories, 0.4 gram of fat, 17 grams of carbohydrate, 13 grams of protein, 174 milligrams of sodium, 4 milligrams of cholesterol, 0 grams of fiber, 45 percent of the USRDA for calcium, 31 percent of the USRDA for riboflavin, and 23 percent of the USRDA for vitamin B$_{12}$.

FIG BARS

A favorite among cyclists and runners because they pack a strong carbohydrate punch and are easy to eat during exercise. Much lower in fat than most treats, fig bars also supply a bit of fiber—not a lot, but more than most sweets.

Two bars have 106 calories, 1.9 grams of fat, 21 grams of carbohydrate, 1 gram of protein, 90 milligrams of sodium, 0 milligrams of cholesterol, and 5 grams of fiber.

GRAPES

Once thought to provide few significant nutrients. Now researchers from the U.S. Department of Agriculture say grapes are a good source of boron, a mineral believed to be important in building and maintaining healthy bones.

A ½-cup serving has 29 calories, 0.2 gram of fat, 1 milligram of sodium, 0 milligrams of cholesterol, and 0.3 gram of fiber.

KIWI

The odd little fruit in the fuzzy brown wrapper proves that good things come in small packages. Each kiwi provides 75 milligrams of vitamin C and 1.7 grams of fiber.

One kiwi has 46 calories, 0.3 gram of fat, 11 grams of carbohydrate, 0.8 gram of protein, 4 milligrams of sodium, 0 milligrams of cholesterol, 1.7 grams of fiber, and 124 percent of the USRDA for vitamin C.

LENTILS

Good sources of protein and complex carbohydrates. They also deliver a good amount of iron, particularly if you're limiting your intake of red meat. Lentils are easier to prepare than other legumes because you don't have to let them soak overnight before cooking. Great on their own, in soups, or as an addition to ground meat.

A ½-cup serving has 105 calories, 0 grams of fat, 20 grams of carbohydrate, 8 grams of protein, 30 milligrams of sodium, 0 milligrams of cholesterol, 5.2 grams of fiber, 12 percent of the USRDA for iron, 7 percent of the USRDA for zinc, and 9 percent of the USRDA for folate.

LOW-FAT OR FAT-FREE CHEESES

These are great sources of calcium, but read nutrition labels carefully: Some of these cheeses aren't much lower in fat than regular counterparts, and they can be high in sodium. Choose one that contains 5 grams of fat or less per ounce.

A 1-ounce serving (Alpine Lace Colbi-Lo) has 85 calories, 5 grams of fat, 7 grams of protein, 85 milligrams of sodium, 20 milligrams of cholesterol, and 35 percent of the USRDA for calcium.

OATMEAL

A good source of soluble fiber, and then some: In a study, adding 2 ounces of oatmeal a day to a low-fat diet significantly lowered subjects' blood cholesterol levels in about four weeks, according to registered dietitian and researcher Linda Van Horn, Ph.D., of Northwestern University Medical School in Chicago.

A ½-cup serving (regular) has 73 calories, 1.2 grams of fat, 13 grams of carbohydrate, 3 grams of protein, 1 milligram of sodium, 0 milligrams of cholesterol, and 2.7 grams of fiber.

ORANGE JUICE

Besides being an excellent source of vitamin C, one 6-ounce glass provides nearly as much potassium as a banana and about 23 percent of the USRDA for the sometimes hard-to-come-by B vitamin folate.

A 6-ounce serving has 76 calories, 0.3 gram of fat, 18 grams of carbohydrate, 1 gram of protein, 1 milligram of sodium, 0.1 gram of fiber, 340 milligrams of potassium, 142 percent of the USRDA for vitamin C, and 23 percent of the USRDA for folate.

PAPAYA

A treasure trove of nutrients. One-half of this exotic fruit provides almost as much potassium as a banana and more than 100 percent of the USRDA for vitamin C. It's also a good source of cancer-fighting beta-carotene.

One-half papaya has 59 calories, 0.2 gram of fat, 15 grams of carbohydrate, 1 gram of protein, 4 milligrams of sodium, 0 milligrams of cholesterol, 1.2 grams of fiber, 395 milligrams of potassium, 158 percent of the USRDA for vitamin C, and about 62 percent of the USRDA for vitamin A.

PASTA

Loaded with complex carbohydrates for long-lasting energy, whether you're an athlete or a businessman. Enriched pasta also provides iron and the important B vitamins thiamine, niacin, and riboflavin.

A ½-cup serving has 77 calories, 0.3 gram of fat, 28 grams of carbohydrate, 5.3 grams of protein, 0 milligrams of cholesterol, 1 milligram of sodium, 35 percent of the USRDA for thiamine, 15 percent of the USRDA for riboflavin, 15 percent of the USRDA for niacin, and 10 percent of the USRDA for iron.

POTATOES

Probably one of the most underrated foods. Besides being a powerhouse of complex carbohydrates, a 6-ouncer also provides almost twice as much potassium as a banana, just over one-third of the USRDA for vitamin C, and 66 percent of the USRDA for iron. It's also a good source of copper, which most people tend to be short on.

A 6-ounce potato with skin, baked, has 337 calories, 0.2 gram of fat, 78 grams of carbohydrate, 7 grams of protein, 35 milligrams of sodium, 0 milligrams of cholesterol, 4 grams of fiber, 974 grams of potassium, 38 percent of the USRDA for vitamin C, 66 percent of the USRDA for iron, 70 percent of the USRDA for copper, and 56 percent of the USRDA for vitamin B_6.

SALMON

One of the richest sources of omega-3 fatty acids, which may provide some protection against heart disease. Eating salmon or other ocean fish like mackerel, herring, or tuna twice a week may be enough to reap the health benefits. Fish oil may also fight arthritis, alleviate psoriasis, and reduce high blood pressure. Salmon is an excellent source of selenium, which the National Academy of Sciences says may play a role in cancer prevention.

A 3-ounce serving, cooked, has 157 calories, 6.4 grams of fat, 0 grams of carbohydrate, 23 grams of protein, 50 milligrams of sodium, 42 milligrams of cholesterol, 0 grams of fiber, 40 micrograms of selenium, 42 percent of the USRDA for niacin, and 35 percent of the USRDA for calcium. Most types of salmon provide about 1 gram of omega-3 fatty acids per 3-ounce serving.

SKIM MILK

An excellent low-fat source of calcium and vitamin D—both important for maintaining healthy bones. Research suggests that you have less risk of developing colon cancer with high blood levels of vitamin D than with low levels. But don't turn to supplements for vitamin D: Large amounts can be toxic.

An 8-ounce serving has 80 calories, 0.4 gram of fat, 11 grams of carbohydrate, 8 grams of protein, 4 milligrams of cholesterol, 117 milligrams of sodium, 0 grams of fiber, 24 percent of the USRDA for vitamin D, and 28 percent of the USRDA for calcium.

STRAWBERRIES

Sweet, delicious strawberries are excellent sources of vitamin C and fiber. They also contain ellagic acid, which may prove important in cancer prevention, according to researcher Gary Stoner, Ph.D., director of experimental pathology at the Medical College of Ohio.

A 1-cup serving has 45 calories, 0.6 gram of fat, 11 grams of carbohydrate, 1 gram of protein, 2 milligrams of sodium, 0 milligrams of cholesterol, 2.2 grams of fiber, and 141 percent of the USRDA for vitamin C.

WATER

The most critical nutrient in your body, it's needed for just about everything that happens, and you lose it fast: at least 2 cups daily just exhaling; 10 cups through normal waste and body cooling; 1 to 2 quarts per hour running, biking, or working out. Eight glasses a day is enough for sedentary folks, but if you're physically active, you need more. Drink 8 to 20 ounces of water about 15 minutes before working out. If you run, drink at least 2 cups of water for every pound you lose on your course.

WHOLE-GRAIN CEREALS

Besides providing lots of complex carbohydrates, they're a great way to get fiber in your diet—a prevention measure that the National Cancer Institute strongly recommends. What's more, research suggests that eating a high-fiber cereal at breakfast may curb your appetite at lunch. Read the labels: A cereal should contain at least 5 grams of fiber and no more than 1 or 2 grams of fat per serving. Some cereals that trumpet themselves as being high in fiber actually provide insignificant amounts and may have as much fat per serving as a pat of butter. Don't worry too much about the sugar content. Actually, a bowl of low-fat but sugary cereal with skim milk is a much better antidote to a sweet tooth than a bowl of ice cream or a hunk of fat-laden cake.

—Densie Webb, Ph.D.

Good Snacks

No need to ax the snacks—between-meal munching
needn't be a bad thing. In fact, these snacks
provide a bounty of healthy energy.

••••••••••••••••••••••

DID FAMILIES OF the 1950s really get together at every meal—
Dad in his cardigan, Mom in her pearls—like they did on "Ozzie
and Harriet"? If so, how did they manage that? Weren't there any
tennis lessons, early-morning business meetings, health clubs, soft-
ball leagues, or yard chores? Where did they find the time?

These days, we're lucky if we get to sit down to one bona fide
meal a day, let alone three squares. We've evolved into a society of
grazers, eating a series of mini-meals or snacks every few hours all
day long.

Another symptom of the decline of civilization? Not necessarily.
Grazing isn't such a bad habit. A good snack provides an extrava-
gant bounty of energy for work or workout. Studies of experienced
cyclists show that eating a carbohydrate snack 1 hour before riding
can increase endurance by as much as 10 percent. Eat a piece of
fruit or a bagel to fuel your muscles and keep blood sugar levels
steady.

On the other hand, who isn't familiar with that drowsy letdown
that follows a large noontime meal? Worse still, if you plan to hit the
gym at 6:00 P.M. without eating a midafternoon snack, you'll feel
weak and unmotivated. Try a high-carbohydrate snack 2 hours before your workout. You'll be pleasantly surprised at the difference in
your energy level. Even if you're not working out, eat a lighter lunch
followed about 2 to 3 hours later by a high-carbohydrate snack. Your
alertness will improve.

GOOD REASONS FOR GRAZING

Research also suggests that a midafternoon snack boosts memory power. Tufts University psychologist Robin Kanarek, Ph.D.,
tested college students on memorization, math problem solving,
reading comprehension, and alertness skills approximately 3½
hours after lunch. Fifteen minutes before testing, some of the students ate a 200- to 300-calorie snack, while others had just diet soda.

All performed equally on math and reading skills. But snackers scored an average of 15 to 20 percent higher than nonsnackers in memory and alertness. Dr. Kanarek suggests that a midafternoon snack can boost the energy supply to the brain, improving certain aspects of brain function. "Snacking on something like yogurt or fruit can really help you think more clearly," she says.

Snackers may have healthier hearts than nonsnackers. Large population studies suggest that people who gorge on one or two large meals daily are at increased risk of heart disease.

There's also good evidence that frequent snacking lowers blood cholesterol levels. Researchers from the University of Toronto Medical School compared the effects of a typical three-meal-a-day eating routine to those of a snacking diet by measuring blood cholesterol and body weight changes. Two groups of 40-year-old men ate identical amounts of food. One group followed the typical three-meal-a-day routine; the other ate 17 snacks a day. After two weeks, researchers noticed no changes in body weights between the groups. They did, however, measure an 8 percent drop in total blood cholesterol in the snackers. More important, artery-clogging LDL cholesterol dropped almost 14 percent among the snackers—a significant enough change, if maintained, to lower their risk for heart disease.

The snackers' lower cholesterol values may be explained by a drop in their insulin levels. As this hormone normalizes blood sugar levels, it also boosts cholesterol production in the body. Thus, the lower insulin levels observed in snackers may inhibit cholesterol production.

• •

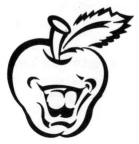

Eve, D.D.S.
Too rushed to brush at the office? Grab an apple after lunch. Apples crunch between the teeth, dislodging food and stimulating saliva flow to counteract plaque, says Elaine M. Parker, former assistant professor of dental hygiene at the University of Maryland.

● ●

SMART SNACKS

With a little advance planning, you can enjoy high-carbohydrate, low-fat snacks.

Choose...	Instead of...	And Save...
2 cups unbuttered popcorn	2 cups buttered popcorn	132 calories, 16 grams fat
1 ounce unsalted hard pretzels	1 ounce potato chips	43 calories, 8 grams fat
2 fig bars	2 brownies, with nuts	84 calories, 10 grams fat
1 Power Bar	1 chocolate bar	105 calories, 19 grams fat
1 bagel	1 doughnut, glazed	42 calories, 10 grams fat
1 cup frozen yogurt	1 cup premium ice cream	133 calories, 22 grams fat

● ●

CAVEAT EMPTOR

Before you dash down the supermarket snack aisle to stock up on chocolate chip cookies, consider that most ready-made snack foods are loaded with fat, sugar, and salt. This is true even of products that no longer use saturated fats like palm and coconut oil. The typical handful of potato chips, for example, derives more than 50 percent of its calories from fat. Don't be deceived by package labels that trumpet "No Cholesterol." The products inside the packages may still be loaded with fat and calories.

Also avoid candy, cookies, and ice cream. They contribute negligible amounts of vitamins, minerals, and fiber, but they do contain lots of calories and may leave you too full for a nutritious meal later in the day.

Take heart, though. This still leaves a wide variety of healthful snacks to fuel your tank. For example, instead of grabbing a 200- to 300-calorie candy bar to perk up your afternoon, bring a package of whole-grain crackers and a can of vegetable juice from home. You'll get a delicious dose of fiber, vitamins, and minerals that's low in fat.

Some other smart snacking ideas:

■ Eat before you get too hungry. Waiting until you're ravenous encourages overeating. Eat every few hours to keep energy levels steady.

■ Keep nutritious snacks handy at work and you won't be as tempted to make a trip to the candy machine. Stash crackers, vegetable and fruit juices, unsalted nuts and pretzels, dried fruit, or unbuttered popcorn in your desk to ward off cravings.

■ Choose snacks with staying power. If you're grabbing a bite after a workout and your next meal is hours away, pick up skim milk and a muffin, yogurt and a bagel, or whole-grain crackers and low-fat cheese. These snacks will also help you bounce back fast.

■ Purchase single servings of packaged snack foods to control portion sizes. It's hard to stop when you're buried elbow-deep in a family-size bag of corn chips.

■ Choose low-calorie snacks if you'll be having a regular meal within an hour or so. Try fresh vegetables dipped in low-cal salad dressing, a small piece of fruit, breadsticks, or unbuttered popcorn.

—Liz Applegate, Ph.D.

Eat to Compete

A few simple nutritional guidelines can boost any athlete's performance. Follow these six rules, and you may find yourself breaking new ground.

•••••••••••••••••••••

TO THE ATHLETE, food can be a friend or a foe. What you eat today will bear on how well you perform tomorrow and the next day. Even the best diet isn't a substitute for talent and training, but the right foods will help you make the most of what you've got.

Unfortunately, good intentions tend to break down at moments of crisis. As you stare at the menu in a restaurant, you can't remember what's better for you than what else, let alone why. At times like these, the whole business of trying to eat right begins to seem like an abstract, obscure nuisance. If everyone else at the table orders steak with béarnaise sauce, "Me, too" is simpler than trying to mentally call up charts and graphs of calories and fat grams.

Forget trying to grasp and apply the complicated chemistry of metabolism, and instead memorize these six rules. If you can remember to use them, you'll be able to choose the right foods to eat, even under difficult circumstances.

Rule 1: Eat protein for strength, carbohydrates for endurance. The basic concept behind your food choices is that food is fuel. An athlete eats to build strength and endurance. Eat high-protein foods for more power, complex carbohydrates for stamina. Quality protein comes from meats and fish, complex carbohydrates from plants. Eat them both.

Rule 2: Two-thirds carbohydrates, one-third protein. Now for the technical stuff. Rule 2 is actually the rule of threes. Imagine that your plate is divided into three equal areas. By volume, two-thirds of your plate should be covered by complex carbohydrates, one-third by your protein item. Of course, you should also eat your vegetables, but you and your mom can discuss that elsewhere.

Rule 3: Eat white. Life is difficult enough without having to make technical food choices at socially sensitive moments, so memorize Rule 3 and eat foods that are white or tan. With minimal rational thought, this rule will result in a diet of potatoes, brown rice, grains, pasta, and cereals (all complex carbohydrates), as well as fish and chicken. Forget cream sauces. The chef is trying to kill you.

Rule 4: In near-terminal fatigue, remember potatoes. The fourth rule is for use when you're too tired to think, let alone cook: Nuke a spud. A baked potato can be produced in 5 minutes in your

• •

HEAVY HITTERS

The top ten sources of protein and carbohydrates:

Protein		Carbohydrates	
Lean meats	Yogurt	Potatoes	Lentils
Poultry	Nuts	Breads	Cereals
Fish	Beans	Rice	Beans
Tofu	Skim milk	Pasta	Corn
Cheese	Lentils	Fruits	Peas

• •

microwave. Top it with salsa, vegetarian chili, or low-fat yogurt. The potato is an athlete's best friend, chock-full of complex carbohydrates, cheap, quick, and easy to cook. If you don't sabotage its innocence with butter and sour cream, a potato contains no fat. While the potato cooks, make yourself a salad and you'll have a meal that provides you with both the building blocks of athletic excellence and the Recommended Dietary Allowance (RDA) of moral superiority.

Rule 5: Put light food on a dark plate for visual relief. The above dietary plan has one drawback: It makes for a dull meal and a boring lifestyle, which leads us to Rule 5. A gleaming black plate will make your white dinner look snazzy, even art deco, sort of. Add a few green vegetables ornamentally, for your mother's sake.

Rule 6: Give it a rest sometimes. When your tolerance for eating right flags, give it a break. A diet is not a religion. Know the rules and follow them when you can, but don't be too hard on yourself if you feel like blowing it all off once in a while.

See you at the finish line.

—Anne Robinson

A New Look
at the Four Food Groups

A group of respected doctors wants to send animal products out to pasture. Is this good horse sense?

••••••••••••••••••••

REMEMBER THE FOUR Food Groups? Meat. Dairy products. Produce. Grains. Since their introduction in 1956, the FFGs were the nutritional equivalent of the Ten Commandments and the Pledge of Allegiance all rolled into one. Eating out of each group every day was supposed to be the ticket to good health.

But if the Physicians Committee for Responsible Medicine—a doctors' group that promotes preventive medicine—has its way, the

Four Food Groups are going to get a whole new look. Grains stay. So do fruits and vegetables, but each one becomes a separate group. So that's three food groups. And the fourth? Legumes. That's right—beans.

Where's the beef (and pork, lamb, and fish)? And where's the milk? On this chart, the two classic cornerstones of the American diet are missing.

"The New Four Food Groups does not say you should never eat meat or dairy products," says Neal Barnard, M.D., president of the Physicians Committee. "What it is saying is that they should be considered options, not essentials."

PLANT FOODS—FRONT AND CENTER

Who are these subversives who want to sweep away two of the revered fundamentals of our way of eating?

Well, the meat and dairy industries are likely to say they are a radical fringe group. True, the members of the Physicians Committee *may* be a bit ahead of the rest of their colleagues, but they have some solid reasons for putting plant foods front and center in the revamped Four Food Groups.

"We considered 1990 a watershed year in learning how what we eat can promote either disease or health," says Dr. Barnard. "1990 saw the publication of two major studies: a long-term study of diet and disease in China by Dr. Colin Campbell, and Dr. Dean Ornish's book on reversing heart disease through, among other things, diet. Both studies showed that a diet based mostly on plant foods, with little or no meat or dairy foods, greatly reduces the incidence and the impact of heart disease and cancer, the two leading causes of death and illness in Western societies.

"The results of these studies, and others done in the last ten years, say to us that the focus of the American diet has got to change and change dramatically," says Dr. Barnard. "It's time to start centering our diet on low-fat, high-fiber foods that promote health and prevent disease. We can't afford to keep basing it on high-fat and high-cholesterol foods that we know can hurt us."

GIVE US THIS DAY
OUR DAILY COMPLEX CARBOHYDRATES

That's why the proposed FFGs make complex carbohydrates the foundation of our daily eating habits. All four of the new food groups—grains, beans, fruits, and vegetables—are high in complex carbohydrates. This reflects the committee's belief that meat and dairy foods are simply not essential.

That's the aspect of the new FFGs that's bound to be the most controversial. It flies in the face of recent dietetic doctrine that fish, poultry, and skim-milk dairy products are important parts of a balanced, healthy diet. Most of the experts we talked to at least recommend eating fish and skim-milk dairy foods. And most consider two servings—but no more—of lean red meat a week perfectly acceptable.

No one, however, disputes the fact that the lower in fat your diet is, the healthier you will be. And the new FFGs should help re-center our diets on low-fat, high-carbohydrate foods.

THE TWO STUDIES THAT MADE THE DIFFERENCE

Dr. Dean Ornish's program for reducing artery blockage with exercise, relaxation techniques, and a vegetarian diet is the *only* regimen ever found to actually turn heart disease around. To reverse heart disease, Dr. Ornish recommends that people eat a high-carbohydrate, *very*-low-fat diet that eliminates all meat and all but a small bit of nonfat dairy foods. Those who want to *prevent* cardiovascular problems are urged to eat only small amounts of fish and skinned chicken, to eliminate red meat, and to use only skim-milk dairy products.

Dr. Colin Campbell's study of diet and health in China may seem a bit more exotic to Americans. Life expectancy in China is much shorter than in the West, largely because the society is poor, semi-industrialized, and mostly agrarian. But the Chinese who beat the terrible odds of dying prematurely from accidents, poor hygiene (which lets killers such as tuberculosis and cholera flourish), and outright malnutrition rarely develop heart disease, osteoporosis, high blood pressure, and cancer. Dr. Campbell thinks it's largely due to their nearly vegetarian diets—the average Chinese not only eats very little meat but uses next to no dairy products—and their physically rigorous way of life.

Several other prominent researchers on diet and disease—including fiber pioneer Denis Burkitt, M.D., and Oliver Alabaster, M.D., a cancer researcher who is also director of the Institute for Disease Prevention at George Washington University School of Medicine—endorse the revamped Four Food Groups.

The Physicians Committee plans to challenge the old FFGs on their traditional turf—the schools—with a new poster that features veggie and grain cartoon characters. And the new FFGs will make an appearance in some new arenas, like restaurants, and in the media as well. "We're doing this because we believe there are strong, scientific reasons for changing our eating habits," says Dr. Barnard, "and because we can no longer wait for the traditional authorities like the U.S. Department of Agriculture to wake up and act on this new knowledge."

For information on obtaining free recipes or the New Four Food Groups poster, write to the Physicians Committee for Responsible Medicine, P.O. Box 6322, Washington, DC 20015, or call (202) 686-2210.

—Martha Capwell

●●

Good Morning Oats

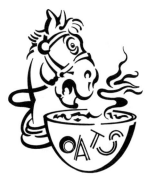

Yes, eating oat bran lowers blood cholesterol, but does the small amount you get in breakfast cereal really help? To find out, researchers in Kentucky studied 12 men with high total cholesterol. All subjects ate the same diet, but some men breakfasted on cornflakes for two weeks, and the rest, on normal-size servings of oat bran cereal—about 2 ounces of cereal, or less than 1 ounce of bran a day. Compared to a diet of cornflakes, the oat-bran diet lowered total cholesterol by 5.4 percent and LDL cholesterol by 8.5 percent— enough to make oat bran cereal a practical tool for lowering risk of coronary heart disease.

Healthy Snacks for Men on the Run

Healthy meals needn't take hours to prepare.
Got a few minutes for some helpful pointers?

• • • • • • • • • • • • • • • • • • • •

WHEN THE AMERICAN Dietetic Association polled men, 82 percent of them said they were concerned about their nutrition. Concern, however, doesn't always translate into actually doing something. Only about one-half of those surveyed said they were making changes in their diet as a result of their concerns.

Why the gap between intention and action? Probably because while many of us want to take better care of ourselves, we can't make a full-time job out of it. (One of those is quite enough, thank you.) If it's going to be a lot of hassle and bother, we'll just have to get around to it later. *Much* later.

Procrastinate no more. Here are 25 quick and simple ways you can get a start toward a more healthful diet.

BREAKFAST

1. Start your morning with a heaping bowl of cereal and you'll likely eat less fat and cholesterol throughout the day—even compared to those who eat something else for breakfast, according to research at St. Joseph's University. High-fiber cereals—ones that contain at least 4 grams of fiber per serving—are better for you, but even sugar-laden kiddie cereals appear to have this fat-curbing effect.

2. Soften butter or margarine at room temperature. Chances are you'll spread your bread with one-quarter of the fat and calories you do when you put it down cold. If you forget, use the microwave.

3. Spread your toast or bagel with fruit preserves or jam, which are fat-free, instead of butter or margarine. You'll save about 4 grams of fat for every pat you don't use.

4. Although whole milk contains only 3.3 percent fat, that measurement is by weight. The true, meaningful measurement of fat is actually percentage of calories from fat, and *49 percent* of the calories in whole milk come from fat. Low-fat, or 2 percent, milk isn't much better: Fully 35 percent of its calories come from saturated fat. But skim milk gets only 5 percent of its calories from fat. In coffee, evaporated canned skim milk makes a decent substitute for half-and-half.

5. Fresh orange juice has more vitamin C than orange juice made from frozen concentrate. Many supermarkets and delis now sell fresh-squeezed, but don't buy more than you can use in four days, since juice begins to lose its vitamin C after it's been opened.

6. Some men just can't face food in the morning. If you're one of them, a good-quality liquid instant breakfast is better than nothing. Look for a product that's low in sugar and that provides one-third of the Recommended Dietary Allowances (RDAs) of vitamins and minerals.

7. If you take vitamin supplements in the morning, you should know how to get the most out of them. Fat-soluble vitamins (A, D, and E) are absorbed best when taken with foods that contain fat. Take them with a glass of milk. Water-soluble vitamins (C and the Bs) should be taken either during a meal or about a half hour before or after eating. Vitamin C should be taken in a few small doses during the day rather than in one big dose.

LUNCH

8. Try canned pink salmon in sandwiches. Salmon is high in potassium and calcium and tastes great with cheese and vegetables. Or prepare a low-fat version of tuna salad by combining a can of drained water-packed tuna with a tablespoon of red wine vinegar and chopped onions to taste.

9. Turn a can of low-sodium broth (beef or chicken) into a quick, healthy meal by adding fresh or frozen vegetables, cooked chicken chunks or diced tofu, fresh or dried herbs and a little sherry, or freshly grated ginger and/or hot pepper sauce. To defat the broth, refrigerate it for a few hours, then skim off all the fat that congeals on the top.

10. Deli sandwiches with all the trimmings aren't the worst things to have for lunch—particularly if you do without the fatty sauces and avoid salt- and smoke-cured meats like bologna, ham, and salami. A case in point: Without sauce, lean roast beef sandwiches are fine.

11. Salad bars can provide the fixings for a nutritious, filling, and low-calorie lunch—or a fat-laden dietary disaster. Here's how to make smart choices:

- Ignore the iceberg lettuce in favor of spinach or romaine or leaf lettuce. They contain more vitamin A and calcium.
- Dip deep into the beans, peas, beets, sliced mushrooms, cucumbers, tomatoes, green peppers, grated carrots, broccoli, and cauliflower. One-half cup of peas, beans, and broccoli gives you over 2 grams of fiber.
- Go easy on the grated cheese.
- If you want a garnish of meat, pick the shrimp, chicken, or turkey. Only 20 percent of their calories come from fat.
- Skip the ham, chopped eggs, croutons, bacon bits, and fried noodles and the salads made with mayonnaise.
- Use no more than 1 tablespoon of dressing, even if there is reduced-calorie available. (The round dippers on most salad bars are the equivalent of 2 tablespoons.)

12. You can make a baked potato flavorful with a few drops of extra-virgin olive oil, soy sauce or Worcestershire sauce, or an herb-and-spice blend. Try this: Mash tofu with a little low-fat mayonnaise, then add curry and herb seasonings to taste.

DINNER

13. Start with a high-carbohydrate food, like a pasta appetizer, bread without butter, or a bean or noodle soup. Studies show that doing so will lessen your appetite.

14. Oven-fried chicken tastes great—without a trace of added fat. Rub skinless chicken pieces with prepared mustard, then coat them with yellow cornmeal. Bake at 450°F for 15 minutes, then lower the temperature to 350°F and bake another 20 minutes or until cooked through.

15. Fish is good food, low in saturated fat and rich in artery-protecting omega-3's. And shellfish lovers should take note that clams, mussels, oysters, and crabs, once suspected of harboring too much cholesterol, have now been put in the clear. But two others, shrimp and squid, still deliver astoundingly high amounts of cholesterol and should be eaten in moderation.

16. We have no beef with beef, as long as it's eaten in moderation. To make sure you get the leanest meat, check the grade. "Prime" and "choice" cuts are the highest in cholesterol. What makes them so tender and juicy is fat. As you descend the meat industry's rating chart, you ascend in health. The "good" and "select" cuts have less fat, fewer calories, and less cholesterol.

Grill your steaks or cook them on a rack or in a slotted pan to let some of the remaining fat drip away. Never rub a steak with oil before cooking it; that will seal in most of the fat.

17. Make your own pizza dough (or buy it ready-made), but instead of the usual toppings, try vegetables like carrots, onions, peppers, and broccoli, either stir-fried in a bit of oil or (better yet) steamed. Top with part-skim mozzarella and bake as usual. Instead of pepperoni, sprinkle on some ground turkey or turkey sausage that you've taken out of its casing.

18. For a fast, nutritious, low-calorie dessert, microwave an apple. Peel the top third to prevent the insides from bursting as the heat expands them. Cover the apple and cook on full power for 3 minutes. Top with low-fat or nonfat yogurt flavored with maple syrup and cinnamon.

SNACKS

19. A frozen juice bar (almost no fat) is a much more healthful cool snack option than an ice-cream bar (15 to 25 grams of fat). If you must have something cold and creamy, have a pudding pop (about 2 grams of fat).

• •

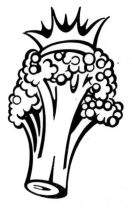

Don't Knock Broc

Forget all that bad-mouthing from the president. Broccoli is the king of vegetables, higher in nutrients and fiber than almost any other food plant. One cup has 164 percent of the Recommended Dietary Allowance (RDA) for vitamin C, nearly one-half of the RDA for vitamin A, 18 percent of the RDA for iron, and more than 20 percent of the RDA for calcium—all for only 46 calories. Broccoli is even believed by some researchers to help prevent cancers of the lung, bladder, and digestive tract.

20. Never eat foods out of their original containers. How many times have you dipped into a pint of ice cream with the intention of having "just a tad," only to find yourself staring at the bottom of the container 15 minutes later? You're much less likely to do that if you dish out the food in a measured portion.

21. Before giving in to that craving for a piece of candy, try brushing your teeth. The sweetness of the toothpaste may take your craving away, and the flavor it leaves in your mouth may make you rethink that handful of jelly beans.

22. Read food labels for clues on sugar content. If the name sugar, sucrose, glucose, maltose, dextrose, lactose, fructose, corn syrup, or any other syrup appears first or near the top of the list, there is a large amount of sugar in that product.

23. Choose pretzels over potato chips or prepackaged popcorn. Pretzels contain about 1 gram of fat per ounce; many chips have ten times that much.

24. An apple a day keeps the droopiness away, suggest scientists at the federal government's Human Nutrition Research Center in Grand Forks, North Dakota. They find that boron-rich foods improve motor skills and boost alertness. Apples and other noncitrus foods such as broccoli, peas, beans, and cabbage are good sources of boron, which also helps the body better retain calcium.

Apples are also good for your teeth. They crunch among the teeth's spaces, dislodging the cavity creators and stimulating saliva flow to counteract plaque, says Elaine M. Parker, former assistant professor of dental hygiene at the University of Maryland.

25. In general, the more the cookie crumbles, the better it is for you. Softer-textured cookies tend to have a higher fat content, with one exception being fig bars. Harder cookies like gingersnaps and vanilla wafers have about one-half the fat of their soft cousins.

Better yet, skip fat-laden cookies and munch on crackers instead. Although some crackers still contain lard, the total amount of fat per serving is much less than the amount in cookies. In general, figure four crackers are equivalent in fat to one cookie.

—*Nick Barton*

All the Taste of Beer

Veteran beer guzzlers rate the nonalcoholic upstarts.
These saintly suds are getting better all the time.

●●●●●●●●●●●●●●●●●●●●●

F. X. MATT II, grandson of the founder of the F. X. Matt Brewing Company in Utica, New York, was showing me around his brewery not long ago. He pointed out a room that, during Prohibition, had housed the dealcoholizing equipment. "Now," he said, "I'm sorry we were so quick to throw it all away."

His regret is understandable. Although Prohibition is gone (hopefully) forever, nonalcoholic beers are making a comeback. There are well over two dozen such brews available today, compared with only five a decade ago. According to Ben Steinman of *Beer Marketer's Insights,* the category was "one of the surprises of 1990—especially after the high-profile introductions of Sharp's (from Miller) and O'Doul's (from Anheuser-Busch)." Miller spent $4.3 million on advertising Sharp's in the first quarter of 1990 (more than on Miller High Life, their regular brand), while Anheuser-Busch doled out $1.2 million in support of O'Doul's.

Nonalcoholic beer clearly is a force to be reckoned with. Still, when *Men's Health* asked me to put together an expert panel for a blind tasting of most of the nonalcoholic brews now on the U.S. market, I was skeptical. As beer expert Alan Eames put it, "Alcohol contributes to the palate experience, to the mouth feel. So as robust as some of the nonalcoholic beers may be, they tend to disappoint. It's like—did I miss my mouth, or what?" Or as American humorist Philander Johnson once said, "The man who called it 'near beer' was a bad judge of distance."

Many of the panelists shared this view going in. But it was clear that nonalcoholic beers are not created equal, because there were some pleasant surprises. (See "How They Fared" on page 60.)

Besides, it doesn't take a social scientist to figure out that the success of nonalcoholic brews (or NABs to the industry) isn't solely about taste. It's about lifesyle. NABs are being marketed as the thing to drink when you want a beer but don't want alcohol—at a business lunch, at a gathering you'll be driving home from, between sets of

(continued on page 62)

• •

HOW THEY FARED

Men's Health rates the nonalcoholic beers.

Brand	Cal./ 12 oz.	Alcohol by Volume (%)	Comments
RECOMMENDED			
Warteck Warteck Brewery, Switzerland	83	0.3	Nice aroma, balanced flavor; a pleasant beer overall
Utica Club NA F. X. Matt, Utica, N.Y.	50	<0.5	Hoppy bouquet, nice head; not enough hop flavor
Haake-Beck Brauerei Beck & Co., Germany	106	<0.5	Nice malt character, pleasant taste spectrum
Buckler Heineken, Holland	75	<0.5	Sweet, malty aroma and taste; good balance
Clausthaler Binding-Brauerei AG, Germany	99	0.44	Fresh aroma, real beer flavor, a bit harsh
Pabst NA Pabst Brewing Co., Milwaukee, Wis.	55	0.3	Clean aroma; nice, balanced flavor; an exceptional lite-type brew
GOOD			
Kaliber Guinness Import Co., Ireland	49	0.01	Sweet, malty aroma, some dullness in flavor
Moussy Cardinal Breweries, Switzerland	50	0.03	Rich color, nutty flavor, mild hop bite, somewhat overpowering malt
Cheers Independent Beverage Group, Hilton Head Island, S.C.	55	0.05	All-American beer, aroma, okay head; sweet, nutty flavor; no aftertaste

• •

Brand	Cal./ 12 oz.	Alcohol by Volume (%)	Comments
Birell F. X. Matt, licensed by Hurlimann, Switzerland	72	0.45	Strong hop aroma, fruity to the max, unbalanced flavor
Pro Dinkelacker Brauerei, Germany	99	0.3	A whiff of the brewer's art, sweet (possibly too sweet), and too hoppy
Texas Select Richland Beverage Corp., Dallas, Tex.	65	0.5	Nice color, sweetish flavor, stale aftertaste
NA Beer San Antonio Beverage Co., San Antonio, Tex.	55	0.2	Delicate hop nose; clean, decent flavor; overcarbonated; stale aftertaste
Goetz Malt Beverage Pearl Brewing Co., San Antonio, Tex.	65	0.3	Clean, sweet aroma; nutty flavor; nice hops; too malty; too thin
Sharp's Miller Brewing Co., Milwaukee, Wis.	74	<0.5	Fresh and clean but overall blah flavor; overcarbonated
O'Doul's Anheuser-Busch, St. Louis, Mo.	72	<0.5	Good aroma, but flavor is absent

DRINKABLE

Brand	Cal./ 12 oz.	Alcohol by Volume (%)	Comments
Hamm's NA Pabst Brewing Co., Milwaukee, Wis.	55	0.3	Okay hop/malt balance, but stale, cardboardy aftertaste
Spirit of the Northwest Pabst Brewing Co., Tumwater, Wash.	75	0.35	Sour, salty flavor
Ziegelhof Brauerei Ziegelhof, Switzerland	58	<0.5	Malt nose, okay balance; mealy, with a rough edge
Kingsbury G. Heileman, LaCrosse, Wis.	60	<0.5	Flat and offensive, lacking in character

tennis—even on military duty. (Moussy and Pabst together donated more than 16,000 cases of their NABs to U.S. forces in Saudi Arabia.) Some guys use nonalcoholic beers as "spacers" between their real beers. In Europe, it's common practice to mix them with regular beer. Among endurance athletes, NABs are sometimes used as part of a postrace rehydration and carbo-replacement plan. Each 12-ounce beer provides 10 to 20 grams of carbohydrate.

Where regular beers have from 4 to 5 percent alcohol, the government requires that NABs contain less than 0.5 percent alcohol by volume. That's not much: Some have even less alcohol in them than fruit juices and soft drinks. Kaliber, from Guinness, is only 0.01 percent alcohol, which, believe it or not, is less alcohol than is contained in a slice of white bread.

To get a brew with virtually no alcohol to taste like beer is no easy task. Joseph Owades, Ph.D., who runs the Center for Brewing Studies in San Francisco when not whipping up new beer recipes for commercial breweries, says there are essentially four ways to do it. The two most common are vacuum distillation and arrested fermentation. The former gets rid of the alcohol after the beer has been brewed; the latter halts the brewing process before appreciable alcohol has formed.

ALMOST SIN-FREE

Since neither of these methods can extract *all* the alcohol, the resulting products can't be labeled alcohol-free. So one way the brews are emphatically *not* being marketed is as drinks for people who can't touch alcohol. "It's not clear how much alcohol will make the difference for an alcoholic," says Chris Larson, manager of aftercare services for the Hazelden Foundation, a drug and alcohol rehabilitation facility in Center City, Minnesota. "But because these brews taste like beer, they might bring back old memories or behavior. That can be dangerous, so we don't recommend them for people in recovery."

Our tasting was held at the Manhattan Brewing Company, where the normal fare is hearty English-style ales made on-premise by brewmaster Mark Witty, one of the judges. Joining us were five other beer and food mavens: Steve Hindy, president of the Brooklyn Brewery; Rick Moonen, executive chef of the Water Club restaurant in Manhattan; Peter LaFrance, associate editor for *Beverage*

Network; Keith Symonds, vice president of the New York City Homebrewers Guild; and Alan Gilbert, an actor and home brewer.

When judgment day arrived, so had fresh samples of 18 NABs, most of the brands on the market. The beers were tasted blind and were rated on a 50-point scale for bouquet/aroma, appearance, flavor, body, drinkability, and overall impression. I cautioned the judges to keep in mind what Jack Kratz, director of sales for Pearl Brewing Company, had advised me: "Comparing NABs to regular beer is like having a Cadillac driver rate a Jeep. They're simply not going to be as aromatic as a regular beer; they're not going to have the body, the fullness, the taste."

On the other hand, that's the way they're being advertised, and there really is no other guide for comparison than one's perception of a decent lager beer flavor. So consistency was what I asked of the judges. This seemed an attainable goal.

As we put the first round of brews through their paces, the prevailing characters of the NABs emerged—malty sweet, cereal-like, light in body and flavor, sometimes fruity, sometimes grassy, sometimes sour, and sometimes, unfortunately, just plain awful.

But there were peaks alongside the valleys. As Witty put it, "The good ones were surprisingly close to real beer. The bad ones were . . . nowhere."

In the end, several judges had beers tied for top honors, so we actually handed out 11 first-place scores: Clausthaler (2), Haake-Beck (2), Utica Club NA (2), Warteck (2), Buckler (1), Cheers (1), and Pabst NA (1). We assigned point values to each beer, depending on how it placed in the judges' individual rankings. These beers rose consistently to the top, with the exception of Cheers, which generally wound up in the middle of the pack, and so all are "recommended" to anyone interested in trying an NAB.

Next there was a drop-off to the larger middle ground of "good" brews, and then another drop between those and the ones at the bottom of the list, which we categorized as "drinkable."

As you'll see in the "Comments" section of the table on page 60, each beer had its adherents and detractors—except Kingsbury, which was roundly disliked by all.

Conspicuous by their absence from the judging were the new high-powered entries in the marketplace, Sharp's and O'Doul's. (Neither of these had reached the Manhattan Brewing Company in time to be included.) To get a reading on these beers, I held an informal home tasting (also blind) a few days later with three friends and my son, all qualified beer drinkers. I put the two beers against ten others. Sharp's barely outpointed O'Doul's, but it seems reasonable to place both in the "good" category.

Afterthoughts? "I don't deny that there are people who like beer, but not its effects," said Hindy. "NABs are a good choice for them."

"I would order one at a bar if I were a designated driver or at a function when I have to drive afterward," said Symonds.

"After the tasting, I went to a reception. I had a Scotch and that was the end of it," said LaFrance. "But I still wanted to drink something, and I didn't want to drink any alcohol, so I had a Sharp's."

Should you try one of these buzzless brews? I have to go back to the advice I gave the panelists. NABs aren't going to deliver the body or flavor of regular beers, but as long as you know that up front, tasting them is a useful experiment: NABs don't have the alcohol, they don't have the calories, and some get surprisingly close to the taste of regular beer.

For Owades, who developed the recipe for Matt's Utica Club NA, the experiment is over. It ended when Sharp's and O'Doul's were introduced in a mega–media blitz to an entire nation of beer lovers ready for an alternative. "Nonalcoholic brews," he said, "are the beers of the future."

—Thomas Bedell

Part 3

MEN AT EASE

The Balanced Life

*Every man—including you—needs a minimum daily
dose of fun. Laughs may be essential to good health.*

• •

To BE A MAN OF robust health, be a man of many pleasures,
advises preventive-medicine specialist and author David Sobel, M.D.
Having fun, feeling satisfied, loving someone, or finding something
deeply agreeable to spend some time on, he says, produces healthy
states in your brain and body. He points to evidence which shows
that cultivating the simple joys of daily life can boost your immunity,
lower your blood pressure, help ward off heart disease, relieve pain,
and maybe even guard against certain types of cancer. "Pleasure is a
prescription for well-being that's filled in the pharmacy of the brain,"

writes Dr. Sobel, coauthor of the book *Healthy Pleasures. Men's Health* talked with him about the role of fun and games in our health.

Q. You begin your book by explaining the Pleasure Principle. Can you sum that up?

A. I've spent the last 20 years looking at what makes people healthy. It turns out that the hardiest, most vital people tend to be pleasure-loving, pleasure-seeking, pleasure-creating people. They enjoy many small daily pleasures, from the sensual to the intellectual to helping others. And this theme of pleasure seems to run through their lives. They *expect* each day to feel good.

This led us to the Pleasure Principle: Enjoying yourself pays off twice. You get the immediate pleasure, and you also get better health.

Q. So doing things that are good for us feels good.

A. It's built into our nature. If evolution wanted to ensure certain behaviors, it could make either the absence of them very painful or the presence of them very pleasurable. We evolved with pleasure centers in our brain to reward us for doing things that fostered survival. For example, our sweet tooth evolved to guide our ancestors toward ripe fruits, which are ready sources of energy and certain vitamins. Our taste for fatty foods, rich in calories, helped ensure our survival during times of famine. Nowadays, while there are exceptions, enjoying food, sex, sleep, friends, work, and family is our innate guide to health.

At the same time, I acknowledge that there are unhealthy pleasures. No matter how much you love to smoke, there's ample evidence that it's not healthy for you. No matter how much you savor the taste of Scotch, drinking a quart a day is bad. The fortunate thing is that *most* of the natural pleasures that we evolved to seek out have added benefits in that they also seem to promote our health.

Q. How is the Pleasure Principle different from mere hedonism, the impulse to do it if it feels good?

A. It isn't all simple selfish pleasures. We found that some of the most enriching things in peoples' lives are selfless pleasures. Whether it's caring for pets, ecology, loved ones, or the homeless, the things that take people beyond themselves are often intensely satisfying and, at the same time, have measurable health benefits.

On the other hand, there's nothing wrong with cultivating sensual and mental enjoyments. Our culture seems to be filled with overindulgence, yet many people don't get their minimum daily requirement of natural sensory pleasures. It's possible for people to get up and shuffle off to work barely noticing the nature around them. To spend all day indoors and never see the sun rise or set. To seldom be touched. To wolf down food and hardly taste or enjoy it. To not listen to natural sounds or pleasant music. This deprivation is at a cost to one's well-being.

Q. Are there any concrete rewards that come from taking time to smell the roses?

A. Research has shown that ordinary pleasures can have dramatic effects on health. A German study found that a group of students who took time out for daily saunas had less than half as many colds over six months as a group that did not. Another study showed that patients recovering from gallbladder surgery spent an average of one day less in the hospital, had fewer complications, and asked for less pain medication if they were given a room that looked out on trees rather than a brick wall.

When investigators piped Brahms into an operating room during surgery, patients needed only half the sedative. Gazing at fish in an aquarium lowered the blood pressure of patients with hypertension. Taking a daily siesta may decrease the risk of heart attack by as much as a third. Being touched can stabilize heart rate—even, at times, for patients who are in a coma. Smelling pleasant scents may improve moods. Getting outside and enjoying the bright natural lighting may help relieve depression. These are all clues that we evolved to seek out natural sensual pleasures.

Q. But the workaday world isn't set up for noontime siestas and soft violins. What practical advice do you have for guys in the business arena?

A. It doesn't take a tremendous amount of time to enrich your life with healthy pleasures. Maybe it's just taking brisk walks outside and really involving yourself in that and enjoying it. It takes only a little more time to really savor your food or notice the smells or aromas around you. If somebody were to say, "I'm going to skip my lunch today and go out and see a funny movie," a lot of people would frown and think he's really goofing off. And yet laughing can raise levels of antibodies that help defend us against colds and respiratory tract infections.

Q. In a balanced life, where do healthy habits, such as regular exercise and eating well, fit in?

A. The latest fitness research suggests that the greatest gains come from modest amounts of daily exercise. I think a balanced view is that health is a tool. That is, it's something we maintain in order to help us achieve something else in our lives.

Q. Do you practice what you preach?

A. Well, I used to play with my son and think about all the work I should be doing instead. Now I understand that playing with him is one of the most productive things that I can possibly do. So the answer is, yes, I'm trying to incorporate this into my life. One of the

• •

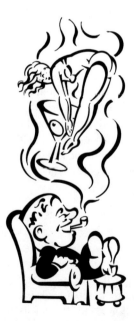

Good Dreams, Bad Dreams

Daydreaming about sex, wealth, and power can be enriching and even healthy—in moderation—according to Ed Beckham, Ph.D., of the University of Oklahoma College of Medicine. But some men go too deeply into their fantasy lives and lose touch with reality. The problem has been dubbed The Walter Mitty Syndrome, after James Thurber's fictional character who copes with life's problems by retreating into his imagination. Daydreams that absorb all one's waking attention are harmful, according to Dr. Beckham, particularly if they are negative, such as prolonged and highly detailed fantasies of revenge or sadism.

principles of healthy pleasures is that none of us is perfect. I don't have to lay that on myself. So I take very small steps. These daily enjoyments not only are the things that enrich my life but actually are some of the best ways to stay healthy.

—John Volmer

Much More Than a Vacation

*Tired of tourist traps? Spend your next
vacation doing something different
and meaningful—like saving the planet!*

• •

VACATIONS ARE A personal kind of thing. You do whatever it takes to get the old batteries recharged. For some guys that involves nothing more than a lounge chair and 151-proof drinks in coconut shells. Others want a break from the day-to-day routine of the job but can't relax sitting on a beach. They need to accomplish something—to climb mountains, explore coral reefs, backpack on wilderness trails, or, perhaps, save the earth.

Put Alex Welles and Tom Grange among that second group. Last year's vacation for Welles, the owner of a real estate company in Seattle, was two weeks in the Soviet Union, helping to build a park. The year before, he hiked the Inca Trail in Peru, not to explore but to pick up trash left by thoughtless foreigners who trek the famous path each year.

"I've always been a socially conscious person," he says. "In the 1960s, I had long hair and granny glasses and went on protest marches. Now I'm in a totally capitalist profession, but I feel an obligation to preserve the beauty I see in the world."

Vietnam vet Tom Grange's return to that country last March was a "self-healing experience." The Boulder, Colorado, police officer went back as part of an Earthwatch study of an almost extinct breed of crane. Its habitat, which had also been a hiding ground for soldiers, was nearly leveled during the war.

"I'd been wanting to go back to Vietnam for a long time, but I didn't want to go strictly as a tourist," he says. "This gave me an opportunity to do something for the country I had helped destroy. I came back from the trip with a good feeling."

An increasing number of men like Welles and Grange are demanding more from their vacations than sun and surf. Through the 1970s and most of the 1980s, a small number of groups offered environmental trips. In the past few years, that number has exploded.

"The number of organizations offering eco-tourism programs has grown at an incredible rate in just the last year," says Mary Pat Sullivan, associate editor of *Tour & Travel News*, a trade publication. "Many environmental activist groups that offered one trip per year for 15 people have branched out to become full-fledged tour operators. They use the revenue to fund their causes. And commercial tour operators are finding they need to include at least one environmental trip because the trips are so popular."

If you'd like to spend some of your time off this year making the world a better place or just learning firsthand what's happening to the environment in other countries, here are some contacts to get you started.

SERVICE TRIPS

Club Med these aren't. For the most part, environmental service trips are lots of work and little play, although you get to do the work in some of the most scenic and remote places in the world. You'll labor shoulder-to-shoulder with scientists, researchers, and environmentalists studying wildlife or restoring ecological systems.

Earthwatch. The granddaddy of environmental organizations. Since 1971, Earthwatch has been matching volunteers to university professors and scientists in 46 countries and 27 states in the United States. Projects include studying glaciers in Switzerland, recording the mating habits of mosquitofish in the Bahamas, preserving the habitat of forest birds in Hawaii, studying coral-reef inhabitants in the Fiji Islands, and tracking kangaroo feeding habits in Australia.

No need to worry that you'll sit idly by as trained professionals do the important work. All projects involve hands-on field research. Participants in a study of endangered leatherback turtles in the Virgin Islands, for example, hike a starlit beach from dusk to dawn for ten nights to track female turtles, tag their flippers, record data on old tags, map locations of nests, and gather eggs to rebury them in a safer spot if the nests are close to the water's edge.

Cost: $25 membership; $800 to $2,000 project fee (includes a portion of the scientist's grant as well as lodging, food, ground transportation). Airfare to site is not included. Earthwatch expeditions are considered scientific research by the IRS, so all expenses are tax-deductible.

Contact: Earthwatch, P.O. Box 403, Watertown, MA 02172; (617) 926-8200.

Journeys. This group runs rugged excursions into Africa, Asia, and South America like the Inca Trail cleanup that Alex Welles went on. It's also involved in trail site restoration, monastery restoration, and a wide range of wildlife protection projects. Trips are graded by the physical demands required: Grade 1, easy hiking; Grade 2, moderate hiking; Grade 3, strenuous hiking at high elevations; Grade 4, technical mountaineering.

Cost: $1,000 to $1,800 (includes accommodations, meals, naturalist guides). Airfare to site not included.

Contact: Journeys, 4011 Jackson Road, Ann Arbor, MI 48103; (800) 255-8735.

Sierra Club. You don't need to leave the country to clean up your act. All Sierra Club service trips are made in the United States, mostly in wilderness areas in the West. Backpacking trips involve constructing or maintaining mountain trails, building bridges over streams or rivers, and revegetating illegal campsites. Sample trips: trail maintenance in Grand Teton, Wyoming; campsite revegetation in Yosemite Park, California; trail building in Grand Canyon Park, Arizona.

Cost: $33 membership; $130 to $255 trip fee. Transportation to site not included.

Contact: Sierra Club, 730 Polk Street, San Francisco, CA 94109; (415) 923-5630.

Volunteers for Outdoor Colorado. Tired of weekends in glitzy Aspen? Most of these projects involve maintaining trails and building handicap-accessible facilities in the Colorado wilderness. Volunteers backpack or stay in campgrounds in mountain parks while working on the projects.

Cost: None.

Contact: Volunteers for Outdoor Colorado, 1410 Grant Street, Suite B-105, Denver, CO 80203; (303) 830-7792.

TRIPS THAT TEACH

Seeing the real thing on vacation beats going to a natural-history museum; for one thing, things move. No classrooms, but you're sure to come home with a degree in environmental awareness.

National Audubon Society. Cruises that care about the environment are the newest wave in eco-tourism, and on this organization's circuit, there's little time for dozing on deck chairs or grazing on gourmet food. Instead, 24 cruises a year feature a smorgasbord of lectures and question-and-answer sessions led by ecology experts. All trips adhere to a seven-point code of environmentally responsible travel, such as prohibiting nonbiodegradable waste disposal from the ships. Sample cruises: Baja whale-watching, Alaskan coastal wilderness, Greek Islands natural history and birdwatching.

Cost: $30 membership; $1,000 to $6,000 cruise fee (depending on ship and accommodations chosen). Airfare to departure point not included.

Contact: National Audubon Society, Travel Department, 950 Third Avenue, New York, NY 10022; (212) 546-9140; fax (212) 832-0242.

American Wilderness Adventures. This group specializes in an up-close-and-personal look at nature with 175 sea-kayaking, rafting, horseback, and hiking trips a year to unspoiled domestic and international locales. All are led by interpretative naturalist guides. A British Columbia sea-kayaking trip will take you to the feeding ground of hundreds of killer whales. You'll also drift by porpoises, harbor seals, sea lions, mink, and river otters. Other sea-kayaking expeditions: Baja whale-watching trip, wildlife photography trip to Kenai Fjords in Alaska.

Cost: Sea kayaking: $650 (British Columbia); $750 (Baja); $1,700 (Alaska). Other trips to $3,000. Airfare to site not included. Between 30 and 40 percent of trip fees is donated to American Wildlands, a nonprofit organization dedicated to river and wilderness protection.

Contact: American Wilderness Adventures, 7500 East Arapahoe Road, Suite 355, Englewood, CO 80112; (800) 322-9453; fax (303) 694-9047.

Oceanic Society Expeditions. Miss Manners would certainly approve of the polite approach to nature viewing practiced by this organization. Guides teach correct animal-viewing skills on 50 trips a year in the Pacific, Caribbean, Africa, and North America. Sample trips: Zaire and Kenya wildlife safari, where participants are taught body language for close-up observation of endangered mountain gorillas; Bahamas dolphin trip, where participants swim with dolphins and observe their underwater behavior.

Cost: $700 to $6,000. Airfare included on some trips.

Contact: Oceanic Society Expeditions, Fort Mason Center, Building E, San Francisco, CA 94123; (800) 326-7491; fax (415) 474-3395.

World Wildlife Fund Expeditions. Learn ecosystem preservation from local conservation experts in South America, Africa, and Asia. Sample trips: safari to the national parks and rain forests of Brazil; natural history trip to Costa Rica.

Cost: $3,500 to $5,800. Airfare not included. A portion of the trip fee supports conservation activities, including preserving rain forests.

Contact: World Wildlife Fund Expeditions, 1250 24th Street NW, Washington, DC 20037; (202) 778-9683; fax (202) 293-9211.

The Nature Conservancy. This ecology group operates over 1,500 wildlife preserves in the United States and offers over 50 field trips per year to the preserves. The emphasis is on outdoor activities rather than structured ecology education. Sample trips: Colorado llama trek; Montana rafting/fishing trip; Virginia barrier islands beachcombing and birding tour.

Cost: $300 to $5,000. A portion of the trip fee is donated to preserving habitats of endangered animals.

Contact: The Nature Conservancy, 1815 North Lynn Street, Arlington, VA 22209; (703) 841-5300.

—Jan Sheehan

15 Roads to Rapid Relaxation

Relax your body. Relax your mind.
Here's how—from deep breathing to sports to sex.

••••••••••••••••••••••

WE ONCE READ AN ARTICLE on ways to unwind that recommended sticking a strip of cellophane tape across your brow so you could monitor your frowns. Right. You'd be the calmest clown at the office. Then there was the book that suggested de-stressing by taking a siesta after lunch. Which makes us wonder: Have these stress experts ever held an actual job?

In the real world, dealing with pressures at work and at home requires an arsenal of *practical* stress solutions. Here are 15.

1. Blow it off. Deep, slow breathing can often calm the fight-or-flight response during periods of big-time stress. Usually, it takes only a few seconds to feel the difference. Simply breathe in through your nose while comfortably expanding first your abdomen and then your rib cage. (Imagine that you're inflating a beach ball inside your gut, through your navel.) Then release the breath through your nose (more slowly than you let it in) and silently say, "Relax."

2. Quick, release. In 3 minutes' time, you can do this to relax your muscles: (1) Sit and close your eyes; (2) inhale, and hold that breath for about 6 seconds while tensing as many muscles as you can; (3) exhale with a whoosh and let your body go limp, then breathe rhythmically for about 20 seconds; (4) repeat twice, and after the third release, relax for a minute, concentrating on a peaceful thought.

3. Make love, not warily. Sex is a good stress reliever. Most people experience a fairly profound relaxation following lovemaking. And since good sex can strengthen a relationship and boost your self-esteem, it's one of the healthiest ways to unwind.

4. Crack up before you crack. A good laugh may break up even teeth-clenching tension. Research indicates that laughter prompts the brain to release endorphins, the body's natural pain relievers. One trick you can use is to keep a tape of your favorite comedian in the glove compartment as an emergency kit for the day when you're late for work, the air conditioner is broken, and the freeway has turned into a parking lot. It works.

5. Get into hot water. "Hot baths are the oldest form of tranquilizer known," says Richard Gubner, M.D., medical director of Safety Harbor Spa and Fitness Center in Florida. He recommends soaking in water that's about 100° to 102°F—in other words, a little warmer than you are—for no more than 15 minutes. A warm shower can help, too.

6. Try some Jacu-pressure. If you have access to a Jacuzzi, try this: Instead of letting the water jets hit you in back, slide down a bit so they pummel your neck and upper shoulders. In combination with the warm water, this gentle massage works miracles. If you can manage it without drowning yourself, let the jets on the other side soothe the soles of your feet.

7. Chill your head, not a cocktail. Instead of an after-work cocktail, try a glass of water or juice followed by 10 minutes of quiet time, preferably in a quiet place with your eyes closed. Explain to those you live with that you need this little reentry period before dealing with leaky toilets, overdue bills, and the fact that Junior broke Mrs. DePietro's kitchen window with a baseball.

8. Walk it off. When possible, don't schedule business lunches. Use lunch as a psychological break, a time to balance out the morning and afternoon. Eat by yourself, and try to concentrate on eating slowly. A noon nap is probably out of the question, but you should be able to take a little walk. People in a study at California State University said a brisk 10-minute walk made them feel less tense for up to 2 hours. "Less tense" in this case didn't mean sedated; they said they felt energized by the walks. Another study found that a 15-minute walk can have a greater calming effect than a tranquilizer.

9. Talk to yourself. It's not a sign you're crazy. In fact, it could help you avoid ending up that way. A private dialogue with your ego is a helpful way to handle stress. "You are less likely to have tunnel vision about a problem when you give yourself a chance to hear, and question, and think out, what you're saying to yourself," says New York psychologist Richard Sackett, Ph.D. In a survey of 208 adults, talking with oneself ranked among the top ten forms of consolation.

10. Don't "awfulize." If you hear yourself saying something like "What a colossal disaster!" on a regular basis, you're probably "awfulizing." If you have to, picture yourself living in Bangladesh during the flood season in order to understand that your kid spilling grape juice on the car seat is *not* a catastrophe.

11. Turn on the tunes and kick back. Some experts say that music for relaxation should be slow, quiet, and instrumental. But don't despair if you get bored with Brahms or feel like punching someone after listening to drippy New Age music. Cheryl Maranto, Ph.D., president of the National Association for Music Therapy, says the two most important characteristics of tranquilizing music are "familiarity and preference." That means Motown or Mingus, Ella or *Exile on Main Street*—whatever makes you happy.

12. Use the gym as a dandy rescue. Regular exercise is probably the single most practical way to throw off tension. Exercising for 40 minutes can reduce stress for up to 3 hours afterward, whereas an equal period of rest and relaxation lowers stress for only 20 minutes, according to John Ragland, Ph.D., of the sports psychology laboratory at the University of Wisconsin. The more stressed you are, the more mellow you'll feel after exercise.

13. Take time to do nothing. It's hard to go from trying to do three things at once to doing nothing at all. But everyone needs some white space on their calendar. "Downtime can be very uplifting," notes Cliff Mangan, Ph.D., a Temple University psychologist. "If you don't have time for yourself and yourself alone, you'll be tense, irritable, and anxious, which is bound to affect others. So in that respect, it's not selfish to be selfish."

14. Give the world permission to be imperfect. "Perfectionism is the world's greatest con game," writes David Burns, M.D., in his book *Feeling Good*. "It promises riches and delivers misery." In a study of more than 700 people, Dr. Burns discovered that perfectionists perfect only distress and dissatisfaction with their careers and personal lives. For all their striving, he found no evidence that they were more successful than their peers. "It's important to recognize that 100 percent is unattainable," advises University of Wisconsin psychologist Asher Pacht, Ph.D. "Settle for 90 percent and recognize that it's a pretty damned good accomplishment."

That's the spirit of compromise you need to keep in mind when tackling stress. But even if you follow every one of these tips and tricks, you'll probably feel wired every once in a while. It's just a natural fact, Jack. The human animal evolved to operate at peak efficiency under a certain degree of stress. Without stress, we'd probably *all* be asleep at our desk by 2:00 P.M. The idea is simply to balance the excess stress with some deliberate mellowness.

15. Call in a pro. If you can't control stress naturally, don't suffer in silence. Talk to your doctor. There are several new drugs that can help control anxiety without turning you into a zombie.

—Michael Busey

Take a Break—To Bake

Saunas offer a hot way to relax. Here are the basics of Scandinavia's favorite pastime.

● ●

THE FIRST TIME I took a sauna was with two neighborhood buddies in the back of a 1964 Pontiac four-door sedan. It was a sweltering mid-July afternoon, and boredom was driving us to creative entertainments.

The challenge: We were to sit inside, windows tight, until someone cried uncle. Heat rose in waves from the macadam driveway as we piled in for self-torture. Sweat beaded on our skin and quickly formed rivers that pooled in the depressions of the vinyl seat. What I remember isn't how long we suffered or who finally gave in, but how unprepared we were for the shock that followed.

We planned to blast out of the car and dive into the Eckerts' pool for a bracing cool-off. But the real surprise came when we opened the door and found that a 90-degree day could feel like ice. We're talking gooseflesh and uncontrolled shivers in the midafternoon sun. The pool felt soothing by comparison. It took several minutes for our internal thermometers to register the pool water cold and the air temperature warm. What a strange sensation!

Who knows, maybe the sauna was invented by such idle creativity; its origin is shrouded in mystery and lore. The Finns argue that they were the first to sauna, although they can't pinpoint the date more accurately than one, maybe two, millennia ago. The Swedes, Norwegians, and Danes make similar claims. In any case, the sauna is as much a part of life in Scandinavia as Monday Night Football is in America. Rural settlers in frozen Norse countries would construct a sauna before tackling less important structures—like houses and barns. For these folks, the sauna is a place where life's worries evaporate like the *loyly*—a Finnish word that means both "steam which rises from the stones" and "soul."

Since my chance exposure to the experience in the Eckerts' driveway, I too have become a devotee. I believe that a winter holiday isn't complete without at least one session. It's a wonderfully hedonistic way to relax in the company of friends or family. There are a few things you need to know to get the most out of your experience.

HEAT TREAT

Saunas differ from other hot baths by being nearly void of moisture, which means a person can bake at higher temperatures comfortably. Ideal heat runs from 190° to 200°F, although temperatures as high as 280° are possible. (The boiling point of

• •

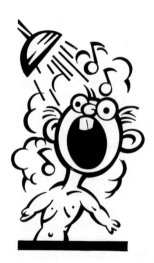

Sing Away Stress

Whether you're trilling Tosca or bellowing some low-down Robert Johnson blues, singing in the shower feels great because it helps relieve stress, says Roger Thies, Ph.D., associate professor of physiology at the University of Oklahoma Health Sciences Center: "Singing forces you to breathe in and out deeply, using your lungs to full capacity," which relaxes the body and can help lower blood pressure. He recommends holding notes as long as possible. Yelling while driving your car has the same effect—but Dr. Thies suggests rolling up the windows first.

water, remember, is a cool 212° by comparison.) Most hot tubs hover at a lukewarm 100°, while steam baths rarely top 120°.

Although purists may swear that a wood-fired sauna is the only true kind, the saunas you'll encounter at resort areas, both here and abroad, are usually heated by electricity. Purism aside, the principle is the same as that for wood-heated saunas: Radiant heat from the main heat source warms not the room but a pile of stones atop the heater. The stones, in turn, make the sauna hot by convection. Convection heat is gentler and more consistent than the furnacelike blast of radiant heat.

The best time for a sauna is after an active day outdoors and before the evening meal. If you insist on a sauna after eating, wait at least an hour: After a meal, blood first shunts to the digestive tract, and if sauna heat is enticing the remaining blood to your skin's surface, it may cause a dangerous oxygen deficiency to vital organs, such as the heart and brain. Presauna cocktails are not a good idea, since alcohol-induced drowsiness could put you to sleep (and if nobody finds you snoozing there, it could be a *very* long sleep).

My favorite après-ski schedule is sauna at 5:00 P.M., a cocktail at around 6:30, and dinner at 7:30 or 8:00. That gives me time to rest, sauna, and catch a second wind before the evening gets rolling.

It's important to warm the sauna and let it "ripen" before entering. That means turning on the heater when you return from skiing, or scheduling a sauna time so your host can fire it up for you. Most saunas have a 1-hour timer switch. Turn it to the maximum setting and you'll have plenty of time to change and relax while it's toasting.

175 DEGREES

The sauna is ripe when the mercury rises to at least 175°F and the humidity drops below 10 percent. High-tech saunas have a thermometer and a hygrometer mounted inside so you can tell when things are just so. In any case, an hour of preheating virtually guarantees a suitable atmosphere.

It's a good idea to drink a glass of water to stave off dehydration before heading in. Since the name of the game is profuse sweating through gaping pores, it's best to remove all sunscreen, makeup, and moisturizing creams or oils, all of which tend to cake on your skin and clog pores.

About clothing: Don't wear any, if possible, but you'd better check out the local customs before bursting in buck naked. (Some resorts avoid any indelicacies by having separate saunas for men and women.) Wearing a loose towel is the next-best thing to bathing naked, with swimsuits a distant third.

Leave certain items behind. Watches and rings not only thwart the bareness ideal, they can sear your skin. Ditto for eyeglasses: Metal frames burn, plastic ones deform. Take out your contacts, because the low humidity can dry them and irritate your eyes.

What you should take to the dressing room is a towel or two, soap, shampoo, shower shoes, a dressing robe, and maybe a bath brush (the modern equivalent of a birch whisk). If there's no bucket and ladle in the sauna, take a plastic cup of water inside for sprinkling the rocks to make steam.

Those are the basics. Now that you're ready for your heat treat, here's a step-by-step guide to the fine points of sauna pleasure.

1. Sit or lie on the lowest bench until you get used to the heat (usually about 5 minutes). Then move up, if you like, to one of the higher benches. Since heat rises, a prone position will provide more even heating than sitting. Relax. Unwind. Avoid unnecessary movements and conversation. Your body will be bathed in a layer of perspiration in a matter of moments.

2. Once you're sweating, sprinkle a little water onto the rock pile. You'll sense an increase in heat and a tingling sensation on your skin. The temperature actually stays constant, but you feel hotter because there's more humidity. The added moisture inhibits sweat evaporation and stimulates your pores to contract momentarily—thus the quivering skin. Don't overdo it with the sprinkles. The idea is to stimulate the skin with humidity, then let the air become dry once again. Too much water spoils the sauna environment and drives bathers out prematurely.

3. For the full treatment, you'll want to try whisking. Truly. So maybe it sounds like some masochistic perversion, but don't knock it until you've tried it. Traditionally, the bather beats his skin with a whisk made from light, leafy birch branches. This stimulates surface capillaries to dilate and heightens the tingling effect begun by the steam treatment. You can get the same effects by rubbing your skin briskly with a rough towel or soft bath brush.

4. Next, step outside and into a warm shower to wash off the dirt and dead skin loosened by perspiring and whisking. Rinse with

• •

WHAT THE DOCTOR ORDERED?

The greatest quality of the sauna, of course, is that it makes you feel so damn good, so loose, so relaxed. It's as if you've cooked the tension right out. While most agree on these feel-good qualities, it's harder to support some of the more tangible health claims that aficionados make. Let's consider a few.

Weight loss. You'll melt off some weight from all the sweating you do in a sauna, but the general consensus is that any change you may notice in the scale afterward should be credited to dehydration—not fat loss.

Cleaning toxins from the body. The theory is that a sauna increases the loss of nitrogen through the skin and speeds up the elimination of waste usually removed by the kidneys and excreted in the urine. That sounds good, but dermatologists say there's no clinical evidence proving that sweating eliminates significant amounts of toxic wastes from the skin.

Improving the complexion. It just ain't so, unfortunately. Heat *irritates* conditions like acne and urticaria, according to skin doctors. There are dermatologists who'll prescribe sauna baths for skin problems related to stress, but that's about as far as it goes.

• •

warm water, rest in the cooler air for a few minutes, then skip to Step 6—or return to the sauna and try Step 5 for the maddest act in sauna lore.

5. Take the plunge. Once you've warmed up again, treat yourself to one of the wildest sensory experiences you can have without breaking the law—the ice plunge. There are several variations: jumping into waist-deep water through a hole cut in lake ice, rolling in a snowbank, hopping into a plunge tank, or taking a cold shower. The secret is commitment. You can't hesitate once you've left the sauna, or your skin will chill slowly and you'll miss the treat. When your skin makes contact with the cold water (or snow), your pores *slam* shut, creating a total body wave sensation.

Don't lollygag in the cold. Either move quickly to Step 6 or hop back in the sauna, warm up, and try the plunge as many times as you like. One caution: If you're bathing in a public facility such as a hotel and plan a naked roll in the snow, make sure the outside door doesn't close and lock behind you. Nothing ruins total relaxation like a naked dash through a crowded lobby.

6. Although it feels relaxing, your body reads a sauna session as a bout of heavy exercise—sweating, elevated heartbeat, systemic surprises—so you should rest afterward. The best dressing rooms have a place to recline on lounges and read the paper, nap, or just zone out. While your pores recover from all that dilating and contracting, let the air dry your skin for 20 to 30 minutes to be sure you've stopped sweating before dressing.

Ideally, you shouldn't take a sauna when pressed for time, but if the need for a quickie should arise, perspiration, washing, and recovery provide the most significant physical benefits. The other steps are mostly for fun.

On a cautionary note, don't take a sauna when suffering an illness, because it adds systemic stress. So forget about "sweating out" that cold or flu. And further, certain people need to approach saunas slowly and cautiously, perhaps with a physician's approval. Folks over age 60 are in a high-risk group for undiagnosed heart disease. The sauna's no place to find out. Children may prefer using the lower benches for a shorter amount of time, because their smaller mass-to-surface-area ratio makes them overheat faster than adults.

Enjoy yourself for however long it feels comfortable. Leave immediately if you feel faint or sense an irregular heartbeat. If that happens, sit in the dressing room and sip water until you recover. Don't try to outlast your pals: Relax, don't compete.

—Don Cuerdon

Swooosh ... Thwack

The aim of archery is to coordinate body and mind.
This chapter targets the details of getting started.

• • • • • • • • • • • • • • • • • • • •

STANDING IN THE Olympic Stadium in Seoul, Jay Barrs could hear his heart thumping above the cheering and applause. One more bull's-eye to win a gold medal, he told himself, drawing back his bow to full tension with a steady grip.

Looking through the sight, his eyes were focused on the target, but he wasn't really seeing it. Effortlessly, he released the arrow and watched as it caught the center spot for the gold.

Archery is a complex and intriguing sport, as much mental as physical. "Being able to hit the target consistently requires focus— the ability to shut out a good deal of conscious thought," says Tim Strickland, an Olympic archery trainer.

AIM WITH THE BRAIN

In sports, this focus is known as "the zone"—an elevated state of psycho-athletic awareness where your body and mind perform their best without any conscious effort. "When you're in the zone, you're still in this reality, but you're capable of watching yourself perform without any evaluation," says Keith Henschen, P.Ed., director of the applied sports psychology program at the University of Utah. He says zone performance is governed by the right hemisphere of an athlete's brain, and it comes into play when the normally dominant analytical left hemisphere cedes control.

• •

Bang, Bang, You're Lead

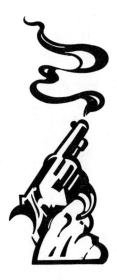

Gun enthusiasts and others who frequently shoot firearms may be accumulating unsafe levels of lead in their blood. Epidemiologists in New Mexico and Colorado found that police recruits who had trained with guns for 1½ hours a week had eight times more lead in their bodies than when they began the course. The cause, say doctors, is the lead dust that's belched from guns. Lead poisoning can lead to lethargy, sore joints, loss of appetite, and other ailments. It takes months for the system to purge itself of the metal. Frequent shooters can protect against lead dust by using copper- or nylon-jacketed bullets instead of the traditional pure-lead rounds.

You don't have to be a world-class competitor to hit the zone. Anyone can do it, and archery is one of the best ways to learn. But first you have to master the basics of stance (straddle the shooting line with your feet shoulder-width apart, your back foot parallel to the line, and your forward foot at a 45-degree angle to it); of anchoring the arrow, at full draw, to a fixed point on your face (and keeping your thumb under your jaw so the string hits your chin and the tip of your nose); and of sighting the target (you never take your eyes off the bull's-eye, and you hold a follow-through position until the arrow hits).

WHERE TO GET STARTED

If you want to take up archery, the way to start is to join a local group. There are clubs in many cities and towns in America; most are members of the National Archery Association (NAA), the country's official amateur archery organization. To locate the club nearest you, contact the NAA at 1750 East Boulder Street, Colorado Springs, CO 80909, or call (719) 578-4576.

Equipment doesn't require a big investment. You can get fully outfitted for $300 to $800, including bow, arrows, and sight. Beyond that, all you need are finger protectors and an arm guard.

Should you find you can hit the bull's-eye with some regularity, you may want to try your hand at competition. There are local tournaments at all skill levels, usually Standard 600 or Standard 900 rounds, where archers launch 60 or 90 shafts from four different distances. Get really good and you can try for the Outdoor Nationals (held every August in Oxford, Ohio), which shoot the same rounds as the Olympic Games.

But the great thing about archery is that you don't have to compete to discover the deep satisfactions of the sport. When it comes to hitting the zone, you have no one to beat but yourself.

—*John F. Hernandez*

Part 4

MAN-TO-MAN TALK

Men Learn the Darndest Things

There are certain rules men live by—as silly as they sometimes are. Why, for instance, can't guys ever stop to ask directions?

● ●

WHEN THE MOVIE *E.T.* first came out, a woman I know was surprised that her husband had shed a tear or two during the scene where the alien munchkin dies. This same guy, see, hadn't so much as misted an eye at *Terms of Endearment,* but a kid's movie got him where he lived.

That's not so odd, I said. Her husband was just following the rules: Guys must stay strong and tear-free through tragedies but are permitted to cry over the death of a pet (and E.T. was essentially Old Yeller from outer space). The only time I ever saw my father cry was the day we buried our dog: As we lowered Duke into a hole in the backyard, he hung his head and bawled.

UNSPOKEN RULES

Men follow a covert propriety—a set of unspoken rules that governs our ways and defines what it is to be male. It's more than just knowing when it's okay for a red-blooded guy to cry; there are dozens of inner directives that tell us how to act like a man.

Where do these bylaws come from? From everywhere: Dad, first-grade readers, coaches, the Hardy Boys, baseball players, Ben Cartwright, older brothers, the Boy Scouts, Ozzie Nelson, and just hanging out with the guys.

Some anthropologists say the codes we follow today were set down way back when men got together to paint bison on the walls of caves. "Many of these behaviors have been selected by evolution," explains Warren Farrell, Ph.D., author of the book *Why Men Are the Way They Are.* "For example, it's a rule that men are supposed to be tough and protect women. This traces back to ancient times, when if women bred with men who were gentle and sensitive, those guys got wiped out by invading tribes. The men who were able to bash in some enemy skulls and save themselves and their women and children were the ones whose genes were passed on."

For modern men, we've compiled a brief list of those unspoken guidelines. These rules look fairly ridiculous on paper, but now that they're documented, you can show them to your wife or girlfriend and say, "See, honey, I'm not the only one who does this stuff . . . "

- On car trips with the family, never ask for directions when you're lost. *Just keep driving aimlessly around, searching for the mysterious Lost Street of the Damned. Navigate by the seat of your pants, like the great explorers of old.*
- But it's okay to stop for directions when driving with another guy. *He won't sit patiently as you pass the same McDonald's for the third time.*
- Inch forward at stoplights to keep up with the guys in the cars on both sides. *It's all about who's out in front.*

- Even if you don't know a hubcap from a distributor cap, never admit you're a stranger to the male domain of auto mechanics. *If your car won't run and you're at a loss for words, try "Could be a cracked ring. Have you checked the compression?"*
- A real man doesn't need the instruction sheet to figure out something as simple as programming his new VCR. *But to cook something as simple as oatmeal, a guy will follow the recipe with the exactitude of a chemical engineer.*
- Don't confess that you know little, and could care less, about a particular sport, especially if it's during the finals. *"Yeah, that Bo, he's really something. What a hook shot!"*
- Never admit you don't understand a political issue. *Opinions are like whiskers: You're not an adult male without them.*
- There's no need to consult *TV Guide* when there's a remote control handy. *Just dive-bomb through all 51 channels, evading commercials like flak, in the never-ending search for a suitable landing spot.*
- If you spill something on the floor, clean it up with a bath towel. *It's unmanly to get down on the floor, so just slop the towel around with your feet.*
- Never pay one of your buddies a compliment. Instead say things like "Who cuts your hair, some guy with a tomahawk?" or "Who is that awesome blonde I saw you with, and what are you going to do for a date once she meets me?" *He'll instinctively get the message that this means you value his friendship.*
- If a man cuts *you* with one of those insults, tell your wife or girlfriend that it hurt your feelings, and you'll come off more sensitive than Phil Donahue. But never reveal it to the other guy. *"Coach, when you said I was a low-life, turd-brained doofus for striking out with the bases loaded, it made me feel small and sad."*
- Never reveal anything about your true, actual, authentic, biological sex life to another guy. *Unless the guy is a urologist.*
- A man should earn as much as or more than his girlfriend or wife. He should be as tall or taller and at least as smart. Naturally, he should be able to outplay her in any activity, from Ping-Pong to chess. *Having met these requisites, he should be liberated enough to be unconcerned about such things.*

- If there are more than two urinals and one is being used, proceed to the farthest available urinal. If a line has formed, maintain proper spacing of at least 3 feet back from any guy using the urinal. *Above all, if nothing happens within 30 seconds, don't just stand there like a geek. Flush the toilet and walk away.*
- When you're in the men's room alone, you needn't wash your hands when you're done. *But if another guy is in there, you scrub your hands like a brain surgeon.*
- If you can't take it (whatever "it" might be), you're not a man. *Maybe you're scared of roller coasters, but if your buddies want to go on one, you'd better gird up your loins and groan through the zero-Gs, or you'll never hear the end of it.*
- Ignore or deny physical pain. *As comedian Billy Crystal reports, "Mike Tyson once hit Trevor Berbick so hard, Trevor did the dance Ann-Margaret did in* Bye Bye, Birdie. *Did he hurt you, Trevor? 'I was stunned, that's all, stunned.' "*
- Never openly display a broken heart caused by a woman or discuss it with other guys. *That's between you, your six-pack, and your collection of Frank Sinatra records.*
- Don't tell another man your deepest hopes or fears. *That's like saying, "How do you like my suit of armor? It's only got two weak spots in it—here and here."*
- If you want to lose weight, don't even think about giving up Ben & Jerry's Chunky Monkey ice cream. *Instead, pull on those running shoes and pound those calories into submission.*
- Every guy should be hip about guns. *Hand an economics professor a Remington, and even if he's never been close to a firearm before, he'll work the action, sight down the barrel, and generally act like a reincarnation of Daniel Boone.*
- If your wife or girlfriend is looking on, flip aloofly through that issue of *Playboy* as if it were a *Better Homes and Gardens* special issue on Tupperware. In a huddle of your peers, pause regularly to utter appreciative comments like "Wow! Check *that* out!" *And if you're alone, study and quantify each curve like a forensic scientist.*
- When shopping with your mate, do not trail her into the women's lingerie department. *Stand clear of those racks of silk-and-lace panties like a jet mechanic would avoid The Whirling Fan Blades of Death.*

—Mark Canter

What All Men Share

*An anthropologist who has studied men
the world over says we aren't so different after all.
See what you have in common with a Masai
cattleman or a New Guinea tribesman.*

●●●●●●●●●●●●●●●●●●●●●

NO MATTER HOW TOUGH it was for you to grow up male in America (yeah, we know, you were the only Italian kid in a Polish neighborhood, or you were the smallest guy on the football team), *nothing* is worse than the hazing teenage boys in Sambia must pass through to earn their manhood, a ritual that involves shoving razor-sharp blades of saw grass up their noses.

On the other hand, boys of all cultures, from the sons of corporate headhunters to the sons of *real* headhunters, are indoctrinated with many of the same male ideals. "I've discovered there is almost a generic criterion of manhood across diverse societies," says David Gilmore, Ph.D., professor of anthropology at the State University of New York and author of *Manhood in the Making.* In his book, Gilmore explores these male role resemblances, stretching from the samurai of feudal Japan to the Samburu of east Africa, from ancient Athens to Athens, Ohio. *Men's Health* asked him to tell what it takes to be a man.

Q. What are the parallels in male images around the world?
A. Manhood is based on being competent in three things. The first is *provisioning.* A real man provides for his wife, his children, and his group—whether he's a Truk fisherman or a Masai cattleman. He has to create a surplus. This is still the big one in Western society; the breadwinner, until the last couple of decades, was almost always male.

The second is *protection.* Defending your clan or country is exclusively a male duty. No nation in the world drafts women for combat. You don't send women of child-bearing age to their deaths if you want your society to go on living.

The third is *impregnating.* In many cultures, having lots of children and wives or mistresses shows that you're a real man.

Q. Why do so many cultures regard true manhood as "a prize to be won or wrested through struggle," as you say in your book?

A. Societies are fragile; they can die away and disintegrate or be taken over by their neighbors. To make the transition from boyhood to manhood, a male must display traits and skills the society needs to survive. Historically, those male roles have involved risk taking, aggressiveness, defense, strength, stoicism, competence, competitiveness, and sexual proficiency. That's where the tests of manhood and the male rites of passage come in. For instance, men are not necessarily warlike—perhaps there's a little bit of the warrior in us because of the hormone testosterone—but it has to be encouraged, shaped by the culture. And cultures do this because *machismo* has helped them survive in many cases.

Q. It sounds as if you're describing a kind of natural selection—the survival of the manliest culture.

A. I wouldn't want to say that without such a model of manly behavior, a culture would surely disappear. But it certainly adds to a culture's strength under conditions of warfare, competition, and environmental struggles, which have been widespread. When those threats disappear, then perhaps you don't need machismo. In fact, that's what I found: Cultures where there is no warfare, strife, or economic competition don't have these same manly ideals and tests of manhood.

Q. What are some of the more unusual male rites of passage?

A. In the highlands of New Guinea, there's an area called the "semen belt" because of a number of cultures with the same peculiar ritual. I wrote about one of them, the Sambia. These people believe that a boy does not develop into a man naturally but must be masculinized by eating the semen of the adults in the tribe.

The Sambia also engage in what is probably the single most painful ritual in the world. The boys are taken into the bush and given stiff, sharp blades of saw grass, which they must shove up their nostrils until the blood gushes. The grown men greet the blood flow with a war cry, for the boys have shown disdain for their own pain and bloodshed—as they will have to do as men on the battlefield.

The Samburu of east Africa are cattle herders. The boys are put through a circumcision rite at the age of 13 or 14. Without anesthetic, their foreskins are cut off, and they are forbidden to move a muscle or cry out in pain while the circumcision is taking place. After this test, they're awarded their manhood, and then they are expected to stand up to lions and defend the tribe from attack. A real Samburu man is supposed to have at least two children and be a good cattleman and provide meat for everyone.

Q. What about in American culture?

A. Boys growing up here are directed mainly to the role of breadwinner and to the values of independence, productivity, competence, and so on. But there are violent subcultures, such as innercity gangs, where males might literally fight to the death to defend their turf.

The rites of passage for American boys are mostly symbolic. You don't actually have to defend your turf, unless you're a gang member. But guys defend their high school's honor in sports, and they take risks in all sorts of ways. Then successful men are expected to channel that drive into college, career, family, and life achievements.

Q. Is there a deeper structure to these cultural resemblances? Is male behavior biological?

A. I don't believe in a universal male or female—but on the other hand, you can't discount 100 million years of evolution. Male and female sex hormones are very different, and they influence us to behave in distinct ways. Culture then takes those biological givens and exaggerates or suppresses them. Some cultures have come close to extinguishing the biological differences between men and women.

Q. We've talked about behaviors and attitudes; what about looks? Are there generic notions about "manly-looking" men?

A. Remember the Bush/Dukakis debates? Dukakis stood on a platform so he wouldn't look small next to Bush. In the United States and all around the world, it's usually tall, muscular men who are the most successful. Their size and strength goes along with the male roles of provisioning and protection. Also, women seem to be more attracted to taller men, so you can include impregnating. Feminists are outraged that men judge women first on the basis of their looks. But turn it around and ask them what they think about weak, skinny little guys . . .

Q. What about cultures that don't fit the pattern? Are there places where manhood is of little importance to men?

A. The two that I came across are the Semai of Malaysia and the Tahitians of French Polynesia. They don't really care about the differences between men and women. There are no tests or rites of passage for the boys. They don't distinguish between a "real man" and an effeminate man—they just don't care. Men and women do pretty much the same jobs. The women are more in charge of child rearing, but both sexes cook, plant, tend animals, and fish. And importantly, both these societies are not warlike.

Q. How did these two cultures cope with warfare?

A. The Semai proudly say, "We run away from danger." They don't believe in bravery. When adrenaline hits and they have the choice of fighting or fleeing, they flee.

The Tahitians long ago enclosed themselves on their bountiful island and did not engage in warfare. They avoid anger and all kinds of aggressive behavior.

Q. What was your most surprising finding?

A. The widespread emphasis on generosity, on male giving; that in most societies, men are expected to produce and give more than they take.

I think the idea that men are privileged and women are under-privileged has been overstated. The fact is, male advantage also carries with it great responsibilities and risks, one of which is to be sent off to war—50,000 men of my generation died in Vietnam. So the critique of the sex roles has to be made with a little more sensitivity to the history of their contributions to the society. I'm definitely not saying that the sacrifices of women should be belittled or ignored, only that the sacrifices of men should be acknowledged and not taken for granted.

Q. What can your research tell the average guy?

A. That it's okay to be a traditional male. That while the traditional gender roles have their limiting aspects, they have provided ways for men and women to complement each other.

Some have argued that because male and female roles are strongly influenced by culture, you can do anything you want with them—even get rid of them altogether. I don't buy that. Just because something is culturally determined doesn't mean it's dispensable. Societies have their needs. You can't just toss out male and female roles that have developed over hundreds of years; the society won't survive.

—*Russell Segal*

Fatherly Wisdom

Looking back, we realize that Dad taught us some important lessons. A survey of men reveals what these lessons are.

• •

WHEN I WAS A BOY of fourteen, my father was so ignorant I could hardly stand to have the old man around. But when I got to be twenty-one, I was astonished at how much he had learned in seven years.

— *Mark Twain*

Fatherly wisdom really does seem to improve with age, but of course, it's *your* age, not his, that makes the difference. Words of advice that did nothing but annoy you as a teenager can suddenly leap across the generation gap and make perfect sense when you reach your thirties. As one man, perhaps less clever but more straightforward than Twain, puts it: "At 17 I got too much of Dad's advice, especially about girls. At 37, I can't get enough."

Part of the problem all along was that Dad didn't always come right out and *say* what was on his mind. What many men remember about their father are examples of his behavior—the way he handled a particular problem or moral dilemma. In his sometimes awkward way, he knew what he was doing.

"Our fathers felt responsible for making men out of us. It was their job," says Ronald Levant, Ed.D., a psychology professor and coauthor of the book *Between Father and Child*. "Men learn life lessons and wisdom from their father, and fathers often teach those lessons by example."

Men's Health interviewed men from across the country—some friends and business acquaintances, some complete strangers—and asked them the most important lesson they learned from their father. Nearly every person interviewed had at least one story to tell; here are some of the best.

My father was giving me a lift to college, and I began griping about how I hated Spanish class so much—not to mention math—and that it made me sick just to think about it. I was about 19 or 20 at the time, and he told me something he'd never talked about before. When he was a young man, he said, working as an insurance sales-man, the boss would line up all the men every morning, as if they were army recruits. He would go down the line and insult and humiliate each and every one of them. That was his way of motivat-ing them. And that was how every day began for my father, week after week, month after month, year after year. But there was a Depression on, and he was glad to have the job, he said. He'd never mentioned this before, because complaining was not in his nature. "If you get through college," he told me, "you won't have to put up with that." I got through college. And a lot of other things.

—Insurance vice president, 51

Dad never got violent or angry; he became "disappointed" when I screwed up. He was my role model, and I wanted his approval. Boy, do I hate "disappointed."

—Advertising executive, 36

On my fourth birthday, my dad took me to Freedomland, a Wild West amusement park in the vast uncharted wilderness somewhere east of the Pecos and west of Fair Lawn, New Jersey. The last attrac-tion of the day was a stagecoach ride, but what began as a pleasant little jaunt soon turned scary when we were bushwhacked by a band of outlaws. They chased us, hooves pounding and guns blazing. Finally, they overtook us, pulled the coach to a stop, threw open the door, and held us up at gunpoint.

Naturally, I assumed they were after my Special Issue Free-domland Souvenir Tricolor Pen, so I did what any self-respecting four-year-old would have done—I cried like a banshee. It was then that my father performed the most remarkable act of bravery I'd ever seen. He looked that gang leader right in the eyes and said, "All right, fellas. That's enough."

To my astonishment, that ruthless desperado looked back at my father and mumbled, "Okay. Sorry, sir." Then he and his cutthroat gang holstered their six-shooters and hightailed it for the hills. The world was safe once again. My dad was a hero. I never forgot the feeling it gave me, and I hope I can make my own son feel that way about me someday.

—Freelance writer, 39

I remember asking him a child's question: "If I were in the street and about to get hit by a car, would you run naked out into the traffic to save me?" He said of course he would. Not just for me, but for a total stranger. I thought about this for a while. I tried to imagine my father the hero, naked and hairy, bounding across the street in the little farm town, saving lives.

—Yoga instructor, 29

The first time I wanted to dump a girlfriend, I couldn't figure out how to do it without bringing down the temple upon my head. I went to my dad and asked him, How do I break up with this girl? How do I tell her that I don't want to see her anymore? "There's no easy way," he said. And as I subsequently found out and have been continuing to find out throughout my life, he was plumb right.

—Wine merchant, 45

The only time Dad ever really *talked* to me was when I was living at home while in college and having my first heavy relationship with a girl. I was coming home late a lot, and as I stole through the front door at 4:00 one morning, Dad came out of his bedroom and took me aside. He said he was concerned about me and we should talk later. We went out to lunch the next day, but he never mentioned the previous night. It wasn't necessary for him to spout off about what was bugging him; just knowing I was keeping him up nights was enough to make me want to mend my ways.

—Editor, 30

My friends and I were out in the woods one day, shooting at cans with our .22 rifles. On the way out we stumbled across a wild turkey, and I impulsively shot it. Since it wasn't hunting season, we got scared and threw the carcass down a steep riverbank. When I got home, my father casually asked what I'd been doing with my gun. I didn't want to lie to him, so I blurted out the tale of the turkey. Without a word, he stood up and went into the other room to get his boots. Then he grabbed two flashlights and said, in a tone that didn't encourage further discussion, "Come on, we're going to go find it." It was cold and dark when we got back into the woods. We searched for nearly an hour, and I was just about ready to plead frostbite when I found the bird. We brought it home, dressed it, and put it in the freezer.

I still love to hunt, but my father taught me a lesson I haven't forgotten. To this day, I've never killed any animal I wasn't prepared to eat.

—Photographer, 40

My dad told me that I should think about having more than one career in my lifetime. "Around 45 you should consider changing your career, maybe not a new field completely, but a major change that will give you new perspectives and challenges and a renewed excitement about life." Shortly after he said this, he followed his own advice and changed careers. As I approach middle age, I'm giving it a lot of thought myself.

—Real estate salesman, 33

My next-door adult neighbor was always picking on me. One hot summer afternoon, I was riding my new Stingray bike and cut across the edge of his finely manicured lawn. He came running out of the front door and yelled, "You little son of a bitch, you ever do that again, I'll break your f—ing neck."

My dad was just coming around the corner in the car with his window open and heard what the neighbor said. He screeched to a halt and, in a quiet but clearly angry voice, said, "Anderson, you ever talk to my kid like that again, I'm going to break *your* f—ing neck." I'd never heard my dad talk like that before, but the neighbor never bothered me again. It made me feel good to know he stood up for me.

—Press secretary, 35

He gave me this warning: "Never quit a job when you're angry." I've been tempted a few times when my ego was bruised or I felt I'd been screwed, but I've always found ways to work things out after I cooled down.

—Hospital manager, 59

My stepfather was a crackerjack car salesman, one of the best. He taught me how to avoid buying a used lemon from a private owner. "Don't talk to the seller when you're looking the car over," he told me. "Kick the tires, open the hood, get under the body, but don't say a word. Most people can't stand the silence—they get nervous and start talking, and what they often blurt out is what's *wrong* with the car. If you run your finger around the inside of the tailpipe for 30 seconds without saying anything, they'll volunteer that the car burns a little oil. It happens every time." The guy was a good psychologist in his own way, which I guess is helpful if you're a salesman. I can't tell you how many junkers I've been spared by using his routine.

—Hotel clerk, 24

He gave me some good advice about those nail-biting periods of anticipation when you're waiting to hear about a job, a lab report, an acceptance to a college. "No news isn't good news," says Dad, ever the bubble-bursting realist. "No news is . . . no news."

Obvious? Maybe. But now when I go through such anxious times, I try not to agonize, play guessing games, or badger the mailman. Instead, as much as possible, I simply get on with my life. As Dad recognized, the news—good or bad—will be the same whether you worry about it or not.

—Bartender, 23

I grew up in a tightly knit community of Cuban Jews where everybody knew everybody else. We had one of everything, and so we had a village idiot, a boy no one ever got to know. One day my father took me aside for the one and only man-to-man talk we ever had, and the core of his concern turned out to be whether I was masturbating and how often. I don't remember any response on my part. But whatever I said apparently was not what he wanted to hear, because *then* he told me that masturbation was very, very dangerous and that there was no telling where it would lead, but one thing was for sure: That slow boy in our crowd was a living example of its evil ways. This was terrifying news for a boy of 12, and for a while afterward, I didn't even allow myself to *look* down there. I think this lasted a week or so.

—Commercial artist, 45

Not all lessons have the intended effect. I'll always remember the time my father spotted two teenage boys in the act of overturning a

Dumpster in front of the apartment building where we lived in New York City. Punks on a lark, they were flinging discarded cartons of papers up in the air and watching the stuff float down like confetti all across the street. My father ran out and seized them by the arms and dragged them into the lobby. Then he called the police. The boys—big, leather-jacketed lugs—wept and pleaded for release. But my father was enraged and determined to carry out this moral lesson to its conclusion. I watched, terrified, from behind the marble balusters on the stairway landing as two policemen came into the lobby and calmly—even gently—escorted the boys out of there. I learned a lesson about civic responsibility that day. I also vowed never to let my father catch me if I got into trouble.

—Production manager, 38

I remember an incident when I was a kid and my father found a wallet. It had a lot of money in it. I thought, "This is great. We have all this money." But my dad called the owner and returned the wallet. I learned a sense of respect for other people's property. I never went shoplifting with my friends—walking out of a store wearing two pairs of jeans.

—College professor, 41

My father repeatedly told my three brothers and me, "Whatever you can conceive and believe, you can achieve." I heard it so often I actually believe it today.

—Carpenter, 31

—Steve Slon and Michael Lafavore

Little Buddies

There are some things about fathering all fathers should know. Topping the list is the importance of simply being there.

• • • • • • • • • • • • • • • • • • • •

WHEN MY ELDEST SON was two years old, he developed a touchingly absurd, endlessly endearing infatuation with garbage trucks. When he would hear the truck lumbering up our little street in Los Angeles, he would literally tremble with excitement. So I'd pick him up and we'd go stand at the curb. The engine would roar and the dumper would clank and the compactor would whine, and sometimes it was so exciting that my son couldn't bear either to look or to look away.

At the time, I just assumed that in the case of my son, this was the way the DNA had fallen into the gene pool, and I gave it no more thought. But then two years later, when my second son reached two, he went through the same wild anticipation at the arrival of the garbage truck. Of course, part of the attraction was the personality of the garbageman himself—he was young and handsome, with a solid build and an impressive black mustache, and he always smiled and waved at the kids. But how much more there was to it I never realized until I recently talked to Mark Gerzon, a trained family therapist and author from Santa Monica. There's a reason so many suburban kids see the garbageman as a hero, Gerzon says: "He's one of the few men that they see working."

Then the light went on. But of course. We fathers, for the most part, are away working in offices. We talk on telephones or sit behind computer terminals. The result is that nowadays, what most fathers do for a living is incomprehensible to their sons. And because of that, something important has been lost.

KIDS NEED VALIDATION

It's hard to put your finger on, says Ken Druck, Ph.D., a clinical psychologist from Del Mar, California, who gives workshops on the father-son relationship. "But I see men walking around in mid-life with a sense of yearning for things that they can't get from their jobs and can't pull from inside themselves. And having listened to thousands of stories in workshops around the world, I'm convinced what the men are missing is a sense of their own identity: a very primitive and deep sense of validation that passes from father to son."

Such validation was easier to come by in times past, when boys could learn what it was to be a man by following in their father's footsteps in a craft or on a farm. And when finally at age 12 or 13, after years of apprenticeship, the boy had earned his chance, the father would climb down from the tractor and say, "Okay, son, it's your turn to plow."

But nowadays the world is too complex. A father can't turn over a Lotus 1-2-3 spreadsheet to his 12-year-old son—the work is too abstract for the boy to imitate usefully (and a lot less fun than driving a tractor). That's one reason why it's so important for boys to have a strong, nurturing, physically active father, says Asa Baber, a Chicago-based columnist for *Playboy*. "A boy wants his dad to be a man. It's the basic plea of the male child: 'Dad, show me how to be a man.' "

ACTIVE DADS, GOOD KIDS

It used to be thought that a father's primary contribution was more financial than emotional. But now it seems the truth may be otherwise. Researchers have discovered that at five months of age, boys who had more contact with their fathers were friendlier with adult strangers than those who had less paternal contact. The infants made more sounds, better liked to be picked up, and got more fun out of playing. Two Dallas psychologists, John W. Santrock, Ph.D., and R. A. Warshak, Ph.D., have further found that boys who live with their fathers after divorce have more warmth, self-esteem, maturity, and independence than boys who live with their mothers.

Basically, says Norma Radin, Ph.D., a University of Michigan professor writing in *Social Work in Education*, "The more time they spend with their fathers, the more socially competent the boys are."

In contrast, when the father is physically or emotionally absent, boys tend to be much more dependent and aggressive and much less compliant. They have more problems in school and in relationships with their friends. They tend to play alone more. "Boys need role models," says Asa Baber. "Boys need fathers. And when they don't get them, they are terrified and embittered."

In an age when so many families are headed by a single parent, it is tempting to believe that fathers and mothers are interchangeable. But it's not true, says Dr. Radin. "Fathers don't mother; they father." Mothers tend to have a verbal, slow-paced style, while fathers have a physical, robust approach.

Furthermore, fathers tend to teach different values than mothers—courage, self-confidence, and a willingness to take risks. Sociologists who have studied fathers and mothers on playgrounds have found that fathers consistently allow their children to roam farther afield, climb higher, and run more risks. "Mothers are wonderful and they provide a safe, secure role model, but boys need someone who is going to encourage them to take risks," says Rick Porter, executive director of the Rainbow River Child Care Centers in Manhattan Beach, California.

TRUST YOUR INSTINCTS

The problem for some fathers is that fear of criticism from their wives, political activists, and self-righteous child psychologists has led them to mistrust their own instincts. So they tone things down around their children. They don't toss them as high, laugh as loud, or even tickle them as wildly. The result, says Dr. Ken Druck, is that they "have given up their natural exuberance and vitality. And that's a tragedy."

The bond between fathers and sons is stronger than the bond between fathers and daughters, says Dr. Norma Radin: "Fathers tend to see their sons' achievements and failures as their own." Everyone knows the bad side of this. That's when you see the fathers with the veins in their necks at a Little League game, screaming at their sons for striking out.

But in a good relationship, the bond between father and son is a two-way street. "Fathers relive their own experience of growing up through their sons," says James A. Levine, director of the Fatherhood Project at Manhattan's Bank Street College. They get to play with Lincoln Logs, run electric trains, play catch, and otherwise act like a kid again. Except this time, the fathers get to do it right.

At the same time, says Dr. Druck, the father teaches his son something he can't learn the same way anywhere else: "What it means to be a man."

—Paul Ciotti

Every Man Needs an Island
Call them hideaways, studies, sanctuaries—
a guy has to have one. Here are some ideas for
finding private space in your life.

•••••••••••••••••••••

AT SEVEN YEARS OLD, I already had a private hideaway. I
dragged an old carpet out of the garage to a musty spot beneath the
raised back porch of our house and furnished my den with a
mildewed armchair, a desk made of cinder blocks and a door, my
entire collection of World War II battleship models, a poster of King
Kong, and a kerosene lamp I didn't dare light. The dampness turned
my Oreo cookies to rubber, and centipedes the size of small alliga-
tors camped out on the deck of my USS *Enterprise,* but until Mom
called me for dinner, I was a content young man.

My search for similar asylums continued through my adoles-
cence and early teens. Every summer I built a new "fort," as far from
home as possible, using any lumber that wasn't already nailed down
somewhere. None would compare to the one I finally managed at
age 14, however: a tree house complete with a bed, sofa, and TV.
There was even room for my two older brothers—and that became
a problem when they found out that there was room for their girlfriends, too. My tree house turned into a penthouse in the time it
took me to climb down to get my guests some potato chips.

Not until after college would I again get anything remotely
resembling what I was looking for, a single room all my own. So
much did I like it that my happiness wasn't even dimmed by the
thinness of the walls—I was regularly serenaded by Jimi Hendrix
from one side and "I Dream of Jeannie" from the other. Alas, I had
to say good-bye to the space less than a year after saying hello to my
future wife.

But the search is all behind me now. This I say with satisfaction
as I lean back in my antique rocker, gaze into the walk-in fireplace of
the 18th-century smokehouse I've converted into an office/retreat—
and try not to notice the bumper of my daughter's Barbie doll
Corvette sticking out from behind the woodbox on the hearth. At 42,
I finally have my space.

GARAGES, BASEMENTS, AND ATTICS

Am I so unusual in my quest for privacy? Eccentric? Egocentric? A "hermit in husband's clothing," as my wife more than once accused?

I don't think so. I like being with my family, but being alone some of the time helps me like them even more. I need my space to work, to ponder, to safeguard the family welfare, to try to bring the big picture into focus.

Talking to other men confirmed my sneaking suspicion that these requirements are not unique to me, that they apply pretty much across the board. My accountant has a private place: a room in his attic where he goes to work on his model trains and listen to old Sinatra records. My lawyer has an area in his garage complete with a pool table, dart board, pinball machine, and refrigerator full of beer. The guy who works on my car has a soundproof room in his basement where he flails away on his drum set and watches the kind of shoot-'em-up videos his wife can't stand. And the list goes on.

"It's as common today for a man to care about his private space as it is for a woman to care about the details of the kitchen," says Greenwich, Connecticut, architect Allan P. Shope. "Men feel they're making a big financial sacrifice when they build a house for the family, so they usually want their own room to be something personal."

Like the one guy who demanded his room have a special door leading to an outside drain, concealed by shrubbery, where he and his buddies could answer the call of nature without having to track into the main house. Like former Gannett Newspapers chairman Allen Neuharth, who built a 216-square-foot tree house on the grounds of his Florida home that has electricity, a toilet and running water, a phone, a built-in desk, a liquor cabinet, and a poker table for four. Like Robert Redford, who has a private "thinking room" at his Utah ranch.

No, I'm not so special. The male animal seems to need privacy—not absolute privacy, of course, but some asylum into which he can retreat from time to time. The big question is, Why? "Men are simply less social creatures," offers University of Pennsylvania psychologist Frank Dattilio, Ph.D. "A woman will call a friend if she has a problem; a man will go sit on the back porch. It's all part of the stoicism we've come to think of as being masculine."

But it's not simply about retreating. It's also about recharging. "The pressures on a man come from many different directions today," says therapist-turned-literary-agent Asher Jason. "They're expected to be cold-blooded as providers but also warm and sensitive as husbands and fathers. I think their need for privacy is a response to this. A man feels a need to refuel so he can keep up the energy required to meet all his obligations. I'm not saying this is true for all men, but I think it's true for many. Their space provides them with an environment to be just who *they* want to be."

John I. Dintenfass, M.D., an assistant professor of psychiatry at Mount Sinai Hospital and School of Medicine in New York City, also likes the recharge theory. "Look at what men put in their private retreats. It's not just the latest wide-screen TV or a state-of-the-art stereo but things very important to them personally—things that help them maintain their identity. This can be important when life's responsibilities begin to be stressful. Men need a space for self-reflection."

PRESSURE SEEMS TO EVAPORATE

If you want to start at the very beginning, consider the male role as it existed at a time when men were dragging home woolly mammoths for dinner, adds Los Angeles psychiatrist Ron Podell, M.D., cofounder of the Center for Mood Disorders. "The male's job was essentially to procure and then to protect the family nest, a function that is apt to have required men to endure extended periods of solitude. His was also the solitary work of hunting and fathering, while the woman was responsible for the more socially interactive duties of child rearing. This might have influenced the development of a more emotionally introverted character structure in the male."

Lest we get too analytical about all this, we should remember one inarguable fact: A lot of us use our retreats for good old-fashioned, bill-paying, Barbie doll–buying *work!*

"I get a second wind when I go to my space," says Bryant Stamford, Ph.D., professor of allied health at the University of Louisville and author of *Fitness without Exercise.* "I can come home up to my eyeballs with bureaucratic bullshit but get a whole new surge of energy the minute I sit down."

"The pressure seems to evaporate when I'm up there," says George Stambolian of his third-story retreat overlooking the ocean on Long Island. "I feel very removed and very focused. I can work for hours up there and have it seem like only minutes."

. . . .

A PLACE OF YOUR OWN: TEN WAYS TO TELL IF IT'S REALLY YOURS

Not unless your retreat meets five or more of the following standards should you feel you have the kind of sanctum you probably need.

1. You go to this space regularly—at least once every two days—and you feel better for the experience.

2. People knock before entering.

3. People generally do not enter if you're not in this space.

4. References to this space generally include your name, as in "I think it's in Bob's study."

5. There is at least one item from your past in this space.

6. There is at least one item that reflects a current interest or hobby of yours in this space.

7. A goal you hold for the future is somehow represented in this space.

8. You would attempt to recreate this space were you to move.

9. Any work you do feels less onerous in this space.

10. You would not hesitate to curse, talk to yourself, belch, or scratch any part of your body in this space.

. . . .

What's so special about working in a quiet place of your own? "There's no interference, no situational static to blur your thoughts," says retired psychoanalyst Herbert Ignatoff, Ph.D., as he lights up a cigar in his richly furnished, wood-paneled study in Cape Coral, Florida. "Our normal working environments frequently distract us in ways we may not even be aware of, but that all disappears when you enter a space that is all your own."

Well, *almost* disappears, I'm thinking as there's a knock on the door from my eight-year-old. "I have a new Ken doll, Dad. Barbie wants to take him for a ride in her Corvette."

—Porter Shimer

Best Friends

Every boy had best friends—where did they all go?
One man courageously looks back.

● ●

NOT THAT I GO AROUND drunk all the time, but still: It is sobering to realize that of the five men whom, from childhood, I have thought of as my best friends, I am actively interactive with only one. One for five: Even in the forgiving arithmetic of big-league baseball, where failure two out of three times is enough to send you to the Hall of Fame, a .200 average is pretty shabby.

Is this my fault? Is it *our* fault? And if the latter, to exactly whom does "our" refer? "Us" as a species? Or just us six guys? Or is the whole thing a nonissue, "best friends" being a term more properly used by kids, young women, and characters in movies? (A freak lab accident has turned Don, a zoologist, into a gibbon. He is confronted by Bob, his best friend. "Don, I'm your best friend," Bob says. "Put the banana down and let's talk.")

In general, men don't talk about having "best friends." At least not in public. They have "buddies," "pals," and so forth, the only manly exception being occasions of betrayal. Thus the classic Mike Nichols and Elaine May sketch, in which an adulterous couple rendezvous—guiltily—in a hotel lobby:

HE: Louise, think how I feel. Will you think how I feel? George is my best friend.

SHE: Your best friend?

HE: He's my best friend.

SHE: He's my *husband.*

At such moments, the term remains useful for its connotations of intimacy and trust—qualities progressively difficult for men to achieve with one another as they trek farther and farther into adulthood, but which youth provides in abundant supply.

Thus the five relationships mentioned above, all of which date from between second grade and my junior year of college. The first two originated in elementary school, in that halcyon interlude between the self-centered heck of young childhood and the girl-centered hell of puberty. With one friend I devised an elaborate culture based upon secret collections: of folk doggerel ("Ladies and germs and bald-headed babies," etc.), of extremely ridiculous secret passwords, of the tiny silver anticlog balls found (at least back then) in Wearever pen cartridges. With the other I pursued a fondness for the Smothers Brothers, science fiction, and *Mad* and traded confidences. With both, sports.

Kid stuff, all of it, but illustrative of the main principle of male friendships: Boys, and men, become friends through shared experience. Women seem able to meet at a party, recognize a kind of common sympathy or mutuality of outlook, and say, "Let's be friends." They even seem able to actually do it. Men, though, need to go through something together, to be paying attention to something external to themselves or their "relationship." Hence the importance of sports (playing, spectating)—not to mention poker, shipwrecks, and armed combat.

TIME AND GEOGRAPHY

But what happens when the shared experience ends? By junior high, these two friends and I moved on to different classes, and then, to different high schools, colleges, careers, cities, wives. (How differently our lives would have turned out had we all simultaneously married the same woman! Yes, and how differently hers would have turned out, too.) I am decisively out of touch with one, sporadically in Christmas card–type communication with the other. I have a more lively and regular exchange with my dry cleaner. And yet I will probably always think of these two boys/men as my original, and therefore most *real,* best friends. Tragedy of the human condition, or routine anecdote of life as we know it?

Maybe both. Such relationships, formed in innocence, must (like innocence itself) inevitably succumb to experience—in this case, brute moving around. And if it's true that "we will always be friends," that statement may include an implicit addendum, similar to the "I'll always love you" murmured by a man and a woman as they break up: ". . . at least, theoretically."

But the end of childhood is no guarantee against impermanency, either. As a university undergraduate, I was best friends with a guy with whom I did everything: attend college, tour Europe, alter consciousness, go to concerts, bare souls, march on Washington.

Since graduation in 1972, we have exchanged, at most, two letters. But then, maybe that's the point: Without such overwhelming, inspiring, and exciting contexts to bring us together, we might have from the start been mere roommates. Which is not to say that a residue of that previous comradeship does not remain; but it feels, as do all those other phenomena, like something that happened back then.

It feels *historical.*

After college I was in a rock band, and I remain good, if somewhat passive, friends with those lads. One, in fact, was best man at my wedding. We speak regularly, get together now and then. He is, for all intents and purposes, my "best friend," but the title is his essentially by default. He also happens to live (relatively) nearby. Is that the key to long-lasting relationships? Geography? But then what are all these fiberoptic telephone systems and fax machines and modems and postal services for, if not to maintain valuable relationships?

Geography, I think, is an excuse. What separates us from former friends is adulthood itself.

What we once got from our best friends we now get from others: companionship from neighbors, world-view mutuality from colleagues, "soul-matesmanship" from wives and lovers. The best friend is thus the general practitioner of youth, replaced in adulthood by specialists. Then, too, our needs themselves change—as is illustrated by my most lamentably ended friendship of them all.

TOUGH ENDINGS

Throughout junior high and high school, my best friend and I performed comedic sketches, wrote a musical, became a team. Our senses of humor were identical. We completed each other's sentences or communicated highly nuanced paragraphs with a phrase. During a dozen years of separation, we stayed in wholehearted, if sporadic, touch.

Then he moved with his wife-to-be to the city where I was living with mine. And the more I spent time with him, the more I felt estranged. Over that 12-year period, I had developed . . . would "a philosophy" be too strong a term? It would. Call it "an outlook," then—one which seemed to me to be at variance with his. I had become something of a leftist, with a satirist's mistrust of consumer

culture. He, meanwhile, had become a middle-of-the-road material-
ist. Gone was the smooth sailing of our teenage sense of humor.
Now our conversations foundered on the reef of different values and
assumptions. My cynical comment about, say, Ronald Reagan
brought no laughing agreement from him; his proud display of a
precious antique elicited from me only polite expressions of
approval. And, of course, we had wives; each encounter featured
eight possible lines of interaction, eight ways to click or not. To my
surprise, when we were together, the air was full of the sound of not
enough clicking.

So I let the relationship die. I stopped staying in touch, felt
guilty about it, and therefore avoided him even more, which exacer-
bated the guilt, and so on. When I moved to a different city, I parted
from him with little ceremony. I felt bad about it then and feel terrible about it now. We had shared not only experience but creativity, a
comedic "take" on the world, in a kind of mutuality found rarely, if at
all, outside professional circles. But the currents of our past relationship simply ran too deep to propel us—or me, at any rate—across
the becalmed gulf of what I, at least, perceived to be the political and
philosophical incompatibility that separated us.

Thus does growing up subvert the very relationships that make
growing up possible. We separate from our parents, whose pleasure
at our being able to do so is usually second only to our own. But we
also separate from our best friends, whom we once took pleasure—
indeed, we took our very identity—in being inseparable from.

—Ellis Weiner

Part 5

THE WOMEN
IN OUR LIVES

Just What Kind
of Mammals Are We?

*Gibbons are monogamous, chimps are promiscuous—
what about humans? Obviously, we swing both ways.
Dr. Frank Pittman suggests the way we should be.*

• •

AS A THERAPIST, one of my jobs is to pick up the pieces of people's lives after they've had affairs. I spend day after day with otherwise sane and successful men who just can't keep their pants zipped, and I begin to wonder if there is some basic flaw in the human animal.

These guys look at me and say things like "The affair felt good, so it must have been okay. My marriage right now feels bad, so the problem must be there. Isn't that logical?" More than one man has suggested something like "Maybe God or Mother Nature has pulled a huge practical joke on us. Maybe women are naturally monogamous and have to get all their security from one faithful man, but men are naturally promiscuous and get their security from running from woman to woman." Or "Maybe this really is hell, and we've been set up to spend eternity in a gender war, with women forever chasing men who are chasing other women."

SWITCH HITTERS

Is monogamy normal? Sure it is. We are perfectly capable of being faithful for a lifetime. Unfortunately we are also quite capable of being unfaithful. There are many forces—physical, emotional, and societal—that can drive a man into another woman's bed. You could almost say cheating on one's wife is as venerable an institution as marriage itself. The trouble is that cheating offers only brief pleasure, and it opens a man's life to a host of unanticipated—and frequently devastating—problems.

A couple of years ago I wrote a book about marriage and infidelity, *Private Lies: Infidelity and the Betrayal of Intimacy*. Since then, I've seen a lot of people, people who otherwise might never have gone to a therapist but who are struggling to put their marriages and lives back together after affairs. Some of them had never taken monogamy seriously and were actually startled when their affairs created problems for them and for their wives. Others had been passionately in love with their wives but went searching for someone new to fall in love with when—as inevitably happens—the first flush of romantic love grew dim. Still others were happily married—the most settled men you'd ever hope to meet—when a chance incident led them astray.

Consider the case of Roy (all names in this article have been changed), who had been in a loving marriage for 20 years. He was a homely man, and Cathy was the first woman who had ever really wanted him. They had great sex, great fun, a great business together, and great kids. Then June sashayed into his life, looking for a job. He didn't offer her one until she already had her hands inside his pants. Roy was surprised at this longstanding fantasy coming true, and he didn't resist.

Unfortunately for Roy, he *didn't* get caught or catch a social disease—that would have been solvable. He treated himself to the full disaster: Roy fell in love. He divorced Cathy and married June, whose hands never again left his pockets. Within a year, his life savings were wiped out and June had run off with another man. By then, he had lost Cathy, his children, and his business—everything in his life. He hadn't known he was unhappily married until June came along. So Roy settled in for a life of low-budget loneliness, but he had—however fleetingly—known "real" love.

DEADLY AFFAIRS

Now, Roy is no different from you or me. It is entirely normal to fantasize about being seduced by a beautiful, mysterious stranger or to dream of having your way with that lithe, single 25-year-old you spot at the gym. So why does acting on the impulse create such a mess for a married man?

The answer is that infidelity sets forces into motion that are completely unexpected, forces that can destroy all the good things marriage can accomplish. In the last 30 years of treating troubled marriages, I've only seen a handful of divorces that occurred when no one had been screwing around. This is important: The likelihood of an established first marriage ending in divorce is minimal unless someone has an affair. Sometimes the affairs took place a long time ago but were kept secret and just drove a wedge in the marriage, slowly pushing the couple apart until they no longer knew one another.

Another client of mine, Stan, has been married 32 years. About 20 years ago, he and his buddies, who were also married, began to seduce other women. It was all very casual, it seemed harmless, and it was a lot of fun. Stan says it was like being 14 all over again and playing on a sports team.

The trouble is, after a few years of this, he felt distant from his wife and uncomfortable around her. His father had had an affair and left his mother. Stan didn't want to be like that. Finally he confessed his indiscretions to his wife, and she—a very understanding woman—forgave him.

Except her forgiveness didn't make Stan feel any better. It made him feel like she was an angel and he was a jerk. So after some time would go by, he'd start looking again for a woman he could feel good with, and all he required was that she be someone he hadn't hurt yet. A cycle was created that Stan couldn't seem to break out of, and it's still going on to this day. Now, finally, his wife is threatening to leave. He's torn between trying to be a good husband—though even having a *good* time with her makes him feel terrible—and running back to his latest lover—a woman he doesn't really *like*. But at least he doesn't feel like a jerk around her.

BAD TRAINING

Why do men cheat when it makes them feel so bad? Simple answer: No one tells them not to.

Of course Roy was attracted to June—anyone would have been. Of course Stan was attracted to the series of women he's fooled around with. The human animal is unlike any other in that it is capable of being interested in sex all month long.

My point is, considering the consequences, being attracted to someone isn't reason enough to screw around. We're attracted to many things. When we see a beautiful car on the street, we want it. When we see a neighbor's house that's beyond our means, we wish it were ours. When a friend's child is doing well in school and our own child is struggling, we may fleetingly wish that the friend's child belonged to us.

But we are perfectly capable—most of us—of reining in these desires. Why? Because they're not healthy for us to act upon, and they're not healthy for society at large. We don't steal the car, burglarize our neighbor's house, or kidnap the child.

Why is it, then, that we *do* feel it's okay—it's a manly thing to do—to screw the woman we want? In my view, it all comes down to training. In America today, we aren't being trained well for monogamy. Several things seem to be going wrong.

First, we're led to believe that we should marry for romantic love. Romance is intoxicating and disorienting, and it takes us away from the real world. But it fades in time. As two people reveal themselves to one another and remain faithful and grow interdependent, the in-love craziness can be replaced by a loving partnership that is a lot saner and nicer. But some people miss the craziness of that in-love state. They feel cheated when it subsides and go out seeking it. Each time they sabotage another relationship, they tell themselves that each woman in turn was just the wrong woman. The problem, of course, is that they are the wrong *man*—too in love with the fantasy of romance to appreciate the reality of love.

Second, we are by nature communal animals. We'd really function best in a large, extended family, where we could have the variety of relationships we need emotionally. A nuclear family of just a husband and a wife and their children is not big enough or varied enough to meet all our needs. The husband and wife frustrate one another and disappoint one another and sometimes bore one another. And when they need an intimate confidant or ally, they don't have a handy relative, so they are tempted to seduce a friend into a special alliance.

Third, nowadays we've got a world full of people who were not raised in families at all and who have no idea how to function in one. Men who grew up with fathers who were busy working, or fighting war, or chasing women, or playing golf, or just hiding from mothers don't have much idea how to be grown men in families. They think the measure of a grown man is that he's old enough and strong enough to run away from Mama. And now they run, too, believing that men who remain domestic and connected to women aren't real men.

Last, there's the religion factor. In my view, it's a shame that religion got involved with marriage. Now that organized religion no longer controls our lives, we tend to ignore it and wipe out its messages. But keeping your marriage together is much more immediate than getting into heaven—or even whether or not you're a good person.

ANIMAL NATURE

Now these are conclusions I've come to from my years as a therapist. But I often wonder whether there is something basically wrong with the human design—especially since it's so clear from where I sit that monogamy is much more likely to make you happy for a lifetime. I've done some reading about the nature of the human animal, and I'll pass some of it along to you.

First of all, it might come as a surprise, but the experts don't really know what manner of animal we are. They're not sure what we would be like if civilization had not come along and cleaned us up and gotten us organized. We are accustomed to thinking of our ancestors as cartoon cavemen with low brows, big clubs, and indelicate seduction techniques, bopping women with clubs and dragging them off by the hair. Is that who we really are, under our Lycra? Or has society changed us right down to the gonads?

We might get some hints by looking at our closest animal relatives. Each of our primate cousins seems to have a different way of mating. If I understand it correctly, the patterns in the wild are something like this: Gibbons are so monogamous that they pair off and stay together in the same tree for a lifetime, fighting to keep anybody else off their limb. Orangutans are confirmed bachelors. They live only one to a tree, come down to mate for a little while, and then go back to their separate trees. Gorillas are polygamous. The big male collects a harem of the much smaller females and then spends his life fighting off the younger males who don't have any females of their own. (Gorillas end up having either no females or so many of them that keeping them is a full-time job.) Chimpanzees are promiscuous. Males and females live in separate bands, but from time to time, the males invade the females and rape them all, then run away again. I may be dramatizing some of the details, but only because I've known people who followed each of those four patterns.

What this shows me is how easily we can shed whatever instincts we have to adapt to the environment—or the culture—around us. It's not that we humans have no monogamous instincts but rather that our instincts are weak and easily overcome. That's not a bad thing. In fact, in many ways, our malleability is the very key to the success of our species. We are so independent of our instincts and so educable that we will become whatever we need to be—and whatever we are trained to be. In modern culture, we are poorly schooled in the values, benefits, pleasures of monogamy.

But monogamy doesn't just feel good and provide a deeper kind of satisfaction than promiscuity; it really is essential to our survival as a species. If we look past the primates at the rest of the animal kingdom, I think we can see why.

Among animals, there are a lot of different behaviors, but to simplify things, let's divide them into two very general categories: herders and nest builders. Most of the herding animals are polygamous, with the males growing big horns and spending all their time and energy battling with one another to see who gets to mate with the females. They don't have much else to do but eat grass for a lifetime. The nest builders have more complicated lives and have more to teach their young. Most of the nest builders are monogamous, and this is the preferred pattern whenever the males have some useful function beyond sperm donation. Nature seems to have decided that babies who someday are going to spend long periods of time raising babies of their own ought to have two parents to teach them.

When monogamous animals are fickle—and even swans, which we think of as being mated for life, sometimes mess around on the side—it can cause a tremendous disruption. After his mate's "affair," the cuckolded male may desert his babies. Ultimately a bird divorce can split the flock.

MARRIAGE IS GOOD FOR SOCIETY

Most societies disapprove of screwing around. And not only that, most of them feel no compunction about intruding in our lives and telling us when to keep our pants on. But there's a reason for that. Societies fall apart when there's no one to raise the children. Promiscuity is the mark of a society that's teetering over an open grave. Dying cultures cease to reproduce, cease to take care of what young they do have, and just screw around until there's no one left to party. Some healthy societies do permit a very controlled kind of polygamy. There are places where you can have a mistress—where, in fact, any man of means is expected to have a mistress—but you cannot divorce. So the marriage—and the man's responsibility to his children—is maintained. There are other places where there is divorce, but infidelity is punishable by death. Extreme, but it certainly controls those promiscuous impulses—all the while allowing a loophole for people stuck in unendurable marriages. There are still other places where you can have more than one wife; but in most cultures where polygamy is allowed, if you want a second wife or mistress, you must first agree to take care of her forever. I've read that only 1 percent of the men in Karachi, Pakistan, take advantage of this option. There, as in most polygamous systems, no matter what a society permits or encourages or requires, most people seek out for themselves some form of monogamy.

I believe this is because we do have a monogamous instinct, weakened though it may be by modern culture. It shows up in the way we fall in love. And it shows up in our jealousy. Here is a core quality of monogamous animals. You don't see promiscuous animals, like dogs and cats, showing jealousy over females. You don't see herding animals getting jealous. Sure, bulls and stallions will fight with other males over control of the herd, but never over any individual female in the herd. Human males and females bond to one partner and become highly agitated when anyone else comes between them. We become obsessively fixated on one another, and what does that fixation signify if not a deep, instinctive need to bond?

The supreme irony is that except at the height of the in-love fixation, the human animal is quite capable of being sexually attracted to others. This feeling—it feels like an instinct to be polygamous—is confusing at best and tormenting at worst. What I tell my clients is that they shouldn't try to deny that they are feeling the attraction. Erotic fantasy is one of life's finest pleasures, and if you don't act on it, you can bring the excitement home.

Looking at the clients I've counseled and the problems they've had with infidelity, I've begun to think the basic nature of the human animal is so monogamous that we stay together forever unless one partner dies or is unfaithful. After a man breaks the bonds of marriage, he may feel so disgusted by their rotten carcass that he can't stand the smell at home. He may go through the motions and still on some level love his longtime partner and the mother of his children, but sexually, he may feel only guilt, shame, and jealousy. He may then go out looking for a woman he hasn't hurt yet and start the whole cycle anew.

The sad part is that we often think it is the problems of our marriage that drive us into the arms of other women. Screwing around is a dumb way to solve any marriage problem I can think of. As a further irony, screwing around is a pretty dumb way to get more sex. Men who have happy, healthy marriages get laid a lot more than serial lovers.

We've got it backward. I've seen men betray some really great wives and some wonderful marriages—because they thought they should, not because they really wanted to. I saw one man who would mess around regularly, while tearfully telling the other women how much he loved his wife. This guy was so sure that real men cheated on their wives, he was *ashamed* by how much he loved her.

Men and women are instinctively monogamous, but with humans, instinct isn't enough. If you've been unfaithful and are waiting for some instinctual power to grab you and push you back into your own bed, forget it. You're going to have to fall back on your intelligence. You can do it, though. Just get out of bed, put on your pants, say good-bye to the nice lady, go home, and tell your wife you're home for good. Then have whatever fantasies you like, and enjoy them to the hilt, and translate them into sexual energy as you screw your wife, and make love to her, too, over and over until you feel really connected again. It won't be difficult. It really is quite natural.

—Frank Pittman, M.D.

What Turns Women On?

Research looks for answers to an age-old mystery. Never mind what you think women like, read what they say.

• • • • • • • • • • • • • • • • • • • •

I'M AN AVERAGE-LOOKING guy. Girls don't faint when they see me, but they don't laugh and point either (at least not unless my fly's open or I have a strand of coleslaw dangling from my chin). It's not so bad, being average looking. You never have to worry that women are only using you for sex; you don't live in constant terror of blemishes; and you rarely get hassled by aggressive crowds of young women confusing you with Tom Cruise.

Of course, all this is easy for me to say, because by some quirky, ribonucleic twist of fate, I happen to possess the one physical trait that appeals to all women, regardless of race, creed, or socioeconomic status: dimples. Don't ask why. Just smile if you have them and leave the rest to the lab people.

But what about the millions of men in the world sadly lacking this whopping genetic advantage? Are there no other physical traits these unfortunate men can fall back on? How can they know if they have what it takes to compete in the terrifying arena of physical attraction?

TANNED, WELL-MUSCLED FOREARMS

After giving the matter a great deal of serious thought, I decided it would be prudent to research this article by interviewing every attractive female in sight. I started by asking my fabulously red-headed and voluptuous hairdresser, Fran, about what she looked for in a man. I expected one of those responses you see in *USA Today:* 43 percent—tush; 30 percent—smile; 20 percent—eyes; 4 percent—nose; and so on. To my surprise, she paused in midsnip and, with a dreamy look, began to rhapsodize about . . . forearms.

"My husband has the nicest forearms. That's one of the first things I notice about a man. Tanned, well-muscled forearms," she said. "Not too hairy; with strong wrists . . . and nice watches. You know, not necessarily super-expensive ones, but not cheap things. I don't know . . . there's something about the way a nice watch sits on a guy's wrist. Especially a guy who really knows how to wear one."

"A guy who knows how to wear a watch?"

"Forget it. It's hard to describe." She resumed snipping.

"No, really. I want to know. This is for science and the betterment of mankind. How's this, for example?" I held out my arm, which I've always felt pretty good about. Besides, I was wearing my favorite watch, a Breitling Navitimer titanium-and-leather. Very jazzy.

"Nice," she said, with the unbridled passion of someone reading the ingredients off a box of Wheatena.

I swallowed my pride and persisted. "But a guy's wrists can't be the first thing you notice. I mean, Quasimodo must've had terrific forearms from years of bell ringing, but if he walked in here for a haircut, you wouldn't be lining up for a date, would you? Now if he had, say, dimples . . . that would be a different story, right?"

"I don't know. You've seen one dimple, you've seen 'em all."

NICE STROKES

Fran's subtle sarcasm notwithstanding, her answer got me thinking. What if men are misguided in their assumptions about what's attractive to women? What if all these guys who have spent hundreds of hours pumping their pecs to look like Roman armor are really getting rejected because of their ankles? How many thousands of sit-ups have guys done to show off their cuts when their fate is being decided on the quality of their kneecaps?

For days and days, I tirelessly examined the intimate sexual thoughts of one beautiful woman after another. It was a tough, demanding job, but . . . well, you know. In the paragraphs that follow are some of the more interesting responses I got.

"I had the biggest crush on this guy in high school," Kris recalled. "He was on the swim team, and what really turned me on about him was watching him do the backstroke."

The backstroke? Not the butterfly? Or the crawl?

"He did those, too," she said. "But it was the backstroke that really got to me. It was such a turn-on. Not the stroke itself, but how into it he was. I guess that's what I find really attractive—seeing a guy doing something he's really into. Seeing him, you know, be what he is."

THE DUDLEY DORIGHT LOOK

The feature that initially attracted Susan to her husband was his "incredibly gorgeous chin."

I'd never met the guy, but a quick scan of the photographs in the room gave me a pretty decent hunch. "Is that him standing over there by the keg?"

"Yes! How did you know?"

"Just a guess," I said, suppressing the urge to point out the amazing resemblance that her husband's "incredibly gorgeous" chin gave him to Dudley Doright of the Northwest Canadian Mounties.

Jane recalled a philosophy professor in college she was crazy about. She was attracted to his pipe—the way he'd speak with it clamped sensuously between his teeth, the burly smell of tobacco, the intense, painful look in his eyes of faraway suffering when he puffed on it. (I wondered if that "painful look" might not have been from the smoke.)

Mary Beth told me about a guy she met over a slab of Monterey Jack at a food co-op in Madison, Wisconsin. He completely charmed her with spiritual talk about organically grown spinach, and she followed him to Oregon to live for the next three months in a teepee.

POPEYE THE SAILOR MAN

After gathering as much research as I could without putting undue strain on my marriage, I collected all my notes and tried to piece together the responses into some sort of perfect male. I combined Fran the hairdresser's husband, Kris's swimmer, Susan's Mountie, Jane's professor, and Mary Beth's kindred-spirit vegetarian. The conclusion should have been obvious to me from the start. Big forearms . . . big chin . . . smokes a pipe . . . and eats spinach—the ideal male is *Popeye the Sailor Man!*

The plain truth is that these women never would have given the other features a second thought if there wasn't an initial attraction to his face. The face is the center for communication. Body language aside, any exchange of information between people, either verbal or visual, has to pass through some part of the face. To put it bluntly, if a woman doesn't find something to like in the face of a beau, the rest of him won't add up to diddley.

So the question becomes: What exactly do women look for in a man's face? There are so many different shapes and sizes, so many varieties. What are her criteria and why? Is she looking for a muscular, strong-jawed he-man or a sensitive, cherub-faced poet? Does she flutter at the sight of cold, steel-gray eyes or melt at the sight of warm, brown, puppy-dog eyes?

A SCIENTIFIC ANALYSIS

Michael R. Cunningham, Ph.D., a professor of psychology at the University of Louisville, has made an in-depth study on the nature of physical attraction. He says that a woman's attraction to a man is based on underlying, and often conflicting, motives, like the desire to nurture and its opposite, the desire to be protected.

Dr. Cunningham suggests that women tend to respond to features in men that trigger a particular balance of these feelings. The ideal male face, he says, is a combination of two opposing types of features: baby-faced and mature. In his formidably titled paper, "What Do Women Want? Facialmetric Assessment of Multiple Motives in the Perception of Male Facial Physical Attractiveness," he describes his efforts, through a series of experiments, to find the correlations between various feature types and physical attraction.

His method was to ask groups of women to rate a variety of individual features in photographs of men in terms of attractiveness, unattractiveness, baby-facedness, and maturity. To correlate the responses, 26 individual facial components in each photograph were precisely measured with micrometers. Included among those

26 components were four separate measurements for the nose (height, nostril width, thickness at tip, and overall nose area), six for the eyes (height, width, vertical eye placement, eyebrow height, pupil width, and horizontal separation between eyes), and three for the smile (area, height, and width).

The results of the experiment showed that an optimal combination of baby-faced and mature features represented the ideal male face to most women. The most consistently desirable features were large eyes, a medium- to smaller-sized nose, prominent cheekbones, a strong chin, and thick eyebrows. The findings also indicated that large eyes and smallish noses were generally considered babyish traits, where sharply defined cheekbones, strong chins, and thicker facial hair (including eyebrows) were perceived as mature traits.

It came as little surprise that large smile areas had an especially noteworthy effect on overall attractiveness, but incredibly, there was no specific mention of dimples in the testing. I pointed this out to Dr. Cunningham, who speculated, rather offhandedly, that dimples might tend to increase baby-facedness but were not likely to tip the scales in and of themselves. I hinted that this was a tremendous gap in his research. He politely took my suggestion under advisement.

It should be noted that the photographs in these experiments were limited to young white males, but according to Dr. Cunningham, the principles of Multiple Motive Attraction apply to all racial types. "Babies in all cultures have large eyes, a small nose, and a small chin," he says. "And you've got to believe that if they find their babies cute, they're also going to find these features to be cute in adults."

What if someone has a huge honker in the middle of an otherwise perfectly featured face? Dr. Cunningham says that various features carry different weights among the individual subjects. According to his findings, for example, a great smile tends to overcome something like a huge nose. Nose size, interestingly, was found to be less detrimental to attractiveness than expected.

What about the other end of the spectrum? Can noses be too small? Dr. Cunningham has yet to find any cultures in which smaller noses are customarily considered unattractive, but he noted, and I'm hard-pressed to disagree, that Michael Jackson may have gone a little too far with that last rhinoplasty.

LOOKING FOR MR. NORMAL

Is there a specific point where features become too large or too small? To answer this, Dr. Cunningham explained the theory of Optimal Discrepancy, which suggests "a curvilinear relation between physical feature size and perceived attractiveness." In plain English, women are attracted to features that don't deviate too far from the norm.

In even plainer English, women like average-looking men, right? Dr. Cunningham said that my interpretation had some merit, mostly if I was looking to give aid and comfort to those with average faces. "What women are looking for," he says, "is something that meets their needs . . . and faces that deviate slightly from the average seem like they may fulfill those needs. So more babylike eyes will make the person look a little more vulnerable and cuddly. If he has just average eyes, he'll look kind of average."

Obviously there's an upper limit on this. You don't want eyeballs that look like the Human Fly. "The most medium guy in our database is not the best-looking guy," according to Dr. Cunningham. "The best-looking guy is the one with the slightly-larger-than-average eyes, bigger-than-average smile, bigger-than-average jaw, slightly higher cheekbones, slightly bushier eyebrows."

What does all this mean to us? How can we put the information we've accumulated here to work in our daily lives?

Well, for one thing, if you have beady little eyes, thin eyebrows, a weak chin, chubby cheeks, and an extraordinarily large nose, you'd be well advised to put some very serious practice time into your smile. More important, we should learn from these findings that our assumptions about how women view us might not be accurate. Maybe the broadness of our shoulders or the thickness of our chest isn't all that critical to a woman, especially if she's the type whose needs lean toward her nurturing side. Then again, those ectomorphs among us with larger-than-average eyes may inappropriately be coming on like a Sensitive New-Age Guy to women who want to be protected. The best advice I can come up with is to try to find the type of woman whose needs fit your needs. How can you tell? Take a shot. If you get rejected, it's a pretty good bet you weren't what she needed.

When all else fails, most of us can take comfort in another of Dr. Cunningham's findings—namely, that women tend to be much less guided by physical criteria than men are. Of course, if that's not enough, you could try to mold yourself into the ideal male—all you need is a little work on your forearms, a corncob pipe, and a can of spinach.

—Jim Goodman

Secrets Men Keep

*There are times to tell and times to clam up—
do you know the difference?
Sex therapist Marty Klein warns that some secrets
can be damaging to a relationship.*

• • • • • • • • • • • • • • • • • • • •

PSSSST. CAN YOU keep a secret? Damn right you can, especially if it's one of your own. We men are notoriously stingy when it comes to revealing what's going on in our heads. We'll talk for hours about the data-retrieval speed of the new PS/2; just don't ask us to share anything really *personal.*

Keeping some things to ourselves isn't necessarily bad. We all need to defend our own little corner of private space. But Palo Alto sex therapist Marty Klein says some secrets, particularly sexual ones, can damage a relationship. "We live in a world that encourages sexual secrets," says Klein, a board member of the Society for the Scientific Study of Sex and the author of *Your Sexual Secrets: When to Keep Them, How to Share Them.* "These secrets don't always protect us or make our lives better. On the contrary, they can hold back the progress of a relationship and distort our sex lives."

Men's Health talked to Klein about when secrets should be revealed and when they're better left unspoken.

Q. When most of us think of sexual secrets, we think of things like cheating on our partner and not telling her. From your book, it's clear that your definition of *secret* is broader than that.

A. Keeping secrets is not just about lying. It's also about withholding information or arranging for people to have the wrong impression about something.

Q. Can you give an example?

A. Let's say a man has a vasectomy and he's perfectly fine about it. Four years later, he starts dating a woman who's interested in having children. She doesn't ask "Did you ever have a vasectomy?"—most people don't walk around asking that. And he doesn't mention it. So by his silence, he allows her to believe he's fertile when he isn't.

Q. I think many people would agree that's not particularly ethical. But your book makes the point that this also hurts him. How?

A. The consequences of sexual secrets are pretty wide ranging. Men who keep sexual secrets always have to fear being discovered. And if the kinds of things that they're hiding involve the way they like to be touched and the way they like to make love, then lovemaking becomes a dangerous enterprise.

This situation leads to a sense of isolation, a distance from your partner. What's really sad is that you never get to know if in fact you are loved for who you really are. There are a lot of men out there saying "Well, she *says* she loves me, but if she really knew what I was like, she wouldn't." Now it may well be that this woman would love him no matter what, but he'll never have the opportunity to find that out.

Q. Is the decision to keep secrets a conscious one?

A. I think that a lot of people don't get the personal space they need. They have to account for all of their time. They feel that they are always under somebody else's inspection. The only way they feel they can create a place where they have a time-out is by creating their own little private world.

A lot of us are not comfortable with closeness and intimacy, and we use sexual secrets to maintain that distance. If you don't want that distance, having sex secrets is going to give it to you whether you like it or not. And if you do want the distance, secrets are pretty handy.

Q. What's the most common secret men keep?

A. It's extremely common for men to masturbate. Among sex therapists, we joke that 90 percent of men masturbate and the other 10 percent are lying about it. A lot of men feel that it is either dishonorable or childish, and they hide this from their partner. What happens is that they feel guilty about it, or maybe they're afraid of getting caught, and they have to do it furtively. This is a real problem. Again, it creates distance—not the masturbating, but the hiding it.

Now I'm *not* telling every man to run and confess to his wife that he masturbates. But in many cases, if he did, it would take a lot of the pressure off.

Q. What about the role of secret fantasy?

A. Again, I don't think that everybody needs to tell all their fantasies. That could be a problem. But just acknowledging to your partner that you think about other people sexually can really be a big relief. I think that we all go around pretending that we never do this. It's obviously not true.

Q. So whether or not you open up about the problem, you have to be honest with yourself.

A. A lot of us, when we make something secret, act as if the thing has stopped existing. That's denying a part of ourselves. For example, suppose you're attracted to someone, and you decide not to tell your regular partner about it. Fine. You do that in order to make life easier for her—and for you. It's not so fine to pretend to yourself that you actually are not attracted to this person.

Q. Where does this need to sweep sexuality under the rug come from?

A. When we were young, most of us were taught that sexuality is bad. We learned that when we got our hand slapped for touching ourselves in public; we learned that when we got our mouth washed out with soap for saying "bad" words; we learned that when our parents were uncomfortable about washing us in the genital area; we learned that when we got punished for playing doctor with Suzie next door. And as a result, we learned that we have to deny our sexuality, hide it—both because we don't want to get punished and because we do want the approval.

Q. Why is there such a cloud of danger around sexuality?

A. The American culture has a conspiracy against sexuality. This is a culture that is suspicious of pleasure. We believe that the human body is fundamentally a dirty object, and that sexual energy is dangerous unless it's channeled in very particular ways. We have more rules about what's right and wrong about sex than we do about almost anything else.

Q. You say in your book that many men have things that they would like their partner to do in bed that they're afraid to ask for. Can you give an example?

A. There are so many examples of things men feel uncomfortable asking their partners for. But let's take a subtle one: Say a man likes oral sex but wishes his partner would do it a little bit differently. She does it, may even be enthusiastic about it, but she doesn't stimulate him in quite the way he likes. If the man doesn't say anything, that's a sexual secret. It's a secret because the man is withholding relevant information.

Q. What's so bad about just enjoying it her way?

A. A lot of men feel that the way *they* like it isn't really okay. They believe it isn't really okay to have a preference. The big thing is normalcy. A lot of men are concerned that maybe it's not normal to want what they want in bed; they fear that perhaps what they desire is so unusual that their partner will not only reject the particular request but will also reject them. But it's important to keep in mind that if you're with someone who loves you, that person wants to please you and wants information about how to do that.

Q. The way you describe it, the fear sounds highly irrational. But aren't there some sexual requests that might send a partner running?

A. Perhaps, but it's extremely common to fear asking for even the most ordinary sexual things. It all comes from an underlying lack of confidence that what we want sexually is okay.

I know when I go to a restaurant, I don't worry "Gee, if I order squid, my wife is going to say 'Get away from me.' " What she'll probably say is "I can't believe you eat squid. I would never eat that. But go ahead and eat it if you want."

We don't, as a rule, worry about whether or not we eat in a normal way. That's partly because we can see everybody eat all around us. If we could know what other people's sexual fantasies are, if we could hear the sounds people make, then we wouldn't have to keep guilty secrets about what should really be nonissues.

Q. I guess it doesn't help that our limited exposure to other people's sexuality usually comes from X-rated videos.

A. Right. We watch Wimbledon on TV, and we don't expect to be able to play tennis like Boris Becker. But when we watch X-rated videos, a lot of us expect to be able to perform that way. Besides, we forget that many of these people's "skills" are due to the magic of editing.

Q. What other common secrets are there?

A. A lot of men have performance anxiety, but they pretend that they don't. What we know about anxiety is that when you talk about it, the anxiety eases. And we also know that people are usually more anxious about things than the situation warrants.

Let's say a man has a few experiences where he doesn't get an erection in the way that he wants to. So the next time he gets into bed, typically he's afraid that he's not going to get an erection. Failing to get an erection is no big deal. But if he's really anxious about it, two things will happen. First of all, it'll be more difficult to get an erection. Second, he won't be able to deal with what's going on in a positive way. For example, if he's really wound up about how this makes him a terrible lover and how he's not a real man, he won't be able to say to his partner "Gee, that's too bad. I wonder what else we can do?'

Q. That's all well and good to say. But after all, there is this woman lying there, waiting for something to happen.

A. In talking with thousands of women over the years, what comes across almost every single time is "I don't mind so much that he doesn't get it up. It's that when he doesn't get it up, he turns away from me."

Q. So in an ideal world, he'd just say …

A. He could say, "Look, it's not working tonight. I hope that's okay. Do you want to talk about it?" Or he might say, "I'm so stressed out. I really want to be sexual with you, but I'm not sure if I can manage an erection. I hope it'll be okay if we do something that doesn't involve intercourse." By discussing the issue, he normalizes it and also gives his partner a chance to say "It's okay."

Q. Isn't it possible that raising sensitive issues will only make things worse? How do you know if it's worth it to open up?

A. There are no guarantees. We'd all like to know "If I do A, my partner will do B." It just doesn't work that way. And furthermore, I don't think conflict is such a bad thing. I think that if you're going to have intimacy, you're going to have conflict. The question is, is it going to be destructive or is it going to be productive?

Q. Why do we expect there to be no conflict?

A. There's a widespread belief that conflict destroys love. People have a hard time understanding that you can be angry at them and still love them. One of the things we can do is to keep reminding our partner *why* we are sharing the information: "I'm telling you this because it's driving me crazy" or "I notice that my sex drive is going down, that I've been avoiding sex with you, and I don't want to do that anymore."

Q. Give an example of a secret that's better kept a secret.

A. Sometimes an extramarital affair is better not discussed. If whatever impelled somebody to do that has been worked out, and there's nothing to be gained from revealing the information, then I'd say just keep it a secret.

As another example, let's say a person has a recurring sexual fantasy about his wife's best friend. Sharing that information could be meanspirited and destructive. Same thing with going into great detail about how she compares to his old girlfriends.

A man needs to ask himself some serious questions about his motives and goals before he reveals secrets about himself. Is it to manipulate, control, or hurt his partner? Or is it honestly to get closer?

If the sharing is for negative reasons, then it's not helpful. Even under the guise of being honest, one can be hurtful. We each know where our partner is vulnerable. The key to all this is to be tender with that spot. Deep down we can tell when revealing a secret is not in the service of either a relationship goal or a personal goal—that's when you don't share.

—Steve Slon

Why Men Cheat

*A psychologist reveals why some men feel
they need a mistress. It's a need, says Dr. Alvin Baraff,
that men are better off without.*

• • • • • • • • • • • • • • • • • • • •

DONALD TRUMP'S peccadilloes may have grabbed all the head-
lines, but he was hardly the only one out there sneaking around.
According to the *Almanac of the American People,* one-third of all
married men stray at one time or another. Other polls have pegged
the number closer to 50 percent. Either way, a lot of husbands
would seem to be having sex with women who are not their wives.

We wondered what's going on in men's lives that tempts so
many of them to wander. For some answers, *Men's Health* turned to
psychologist Alvin Baraff, Ph.D., founder of MenCenter, a psychotherapy practice in Washington, D.C., and author of the forth-
coming book *Men Talk.* Dr. Baraff, who says one out of five of his
clients has had an affair "and for about 10 percent, it's their main
reason for seeking therapy," has heard it all.

Q. Why do married men have affairs?
A. Many times the affair is not just about sex. I recall a client who
lost his job and was feeling very bad about it. His wife was into her
own career and didn't realize how depressed he was. A woman at
his old job was more understanding and lent a sympathetic ear. One
thing led to another and it turned into an affair. But the problem
could be traced back to a lack of communication between him and
his wife.

Many men end up feeling very lonely in their marriage. When
a guy gets married, he often doesn't keep up with the social end of
his life. Then, as his family grows, his wife may have less time to
give him enough attention. The husband can feel left out and start
believing he's only a meal ticket. An affair may be his way of seeking
emotional and sexual attention.

A common cause is that the man is angry with his wife, or she
with him. They're mad and they're not talking about what's making

them mad. Bad feelings are held in and unresolved. Being angry with each other is just the opposite of wanting to make love with each other. So the man will go and find someone outside the relationship, someone who's not mad at him.

That same anger between husband and wife can also lead to the man having a problem with impotence. He may not be able to get an erection because deep down, he's feeling anger toward his wife, but he's not talking to her about it. So he'll have an affair to see if he can get it up, and the odds are that without the emotional baggage, he'll be able to.

Some husbands just aren't getting enough sex. One of my clients, a man in his thirties, was only having sex with his wife about once every two months, and he always had to be the one to initiate it.

• •

Healthy Unions

It should come as no surprise that married men are healthier than unmarried ones. Presumably, we get married because we have the sense to know it's good for us. But just what is it about marriage that's healthy?

Does marriage cause people to lead a healthier lifestyle? Or do healthy people get married? The answer may be yes to both questions, but the combo still won't entirely explain the health benefits married people enjoy.

Researchers at the University of Newcastle in Australia report that among 225,800 residents of New South Wales, unmarried men were between 47 and 120 percent more likely to have a heart attack than the married ones.

Not only that, the married men who did have a heart attack were more than twice as likely as the unmarried men to survive longer than 28 days after the event.

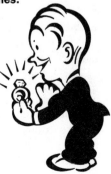

Commenting on the report, Alan J. Goble, a senior cardiologist at Austin Hospital in Melbourne, concluded: "If an unmarried man wishes to prolong his life to the maximum, it may be that he should seek a caring wife."

He started to feel like he was begging, that she was doing him a favor. It became humiliating. He didn't want a divorce, so he had an affair.

Another of my clients, who became impotent with his wife after she constantly refused to have sex, met a woman who approached *him* for an affair. That gave his ego a real boost. He said he never knew that sex could be so enjoyable. He and his lover got divorces and married each other, and it's worked out nicely.

Q. How often do things end that way?

A. It's rare. Another reason for having an affair is to *avoid* a divorce. The guy is loyal and committed to his marriage in nonsexual ways or feels that getting a divorce wouldn't be right for his children. So he gets his sexual needs met through an affair.

Q. So why do men come to see you about their affairs?

A. First, remember that most men *don't* end up talking to a therapist. For those that do, even though they may seem to have reasons for an affair, they still feel very guilty. Not only do they feel they've betrayed their wife and family, but most of the men say they feel they've let *themselves* down. Their self-image is shattered.

After all, most men go into a marriage with the attitude that it's forever. It's only in recent times that we're hearing about prenuptial agreements or so much concern about bailing out if it doesn't work. That hasn't been the tradition.

Q. Do some men secretly hope their wife will catch them?

A. I don't think men *consciously* want that to happen, but if the guilt gets too strong, a guy will often manage to leave some evidence for his wife to uncover. Subconsciously, he wants to take the punishment he feels he deserves. And saying "My wife found out" can help him get out of the affair if he wants to.

One man left a romantic card in his briefcase. His wife found it and confronted him. On the other hand, most wives can sense something is going on, even when the husband thinks he's being clever about it.

Q. What have you heard that has surprised you?

A. I was surprised at how many men are ashamed of themselves. With the exception of *Fatal Attraction,* the way affairs are depicted in books and movies is pretty romantic. They don't usually show the man overwhelmed by guilt.

Something I hadn't given much thought to, until I started hearing it over and over, is how expensive it is to have an affair. Most of the men pay for all the dates and hotel rooms and so forth.

The other surprising thing is how quickly affairs lose their glitter and fun and how soon the men wanted to get out of it. I've heard lots of horror stories about men trying to break off affairs. One client was very high up in a government agency and was having an affair with one of his staff—a very bad idea, but it happens all the time. When the relationship ended, she filed a grievance against him, and he was transferred. In the meantime, his wife found out about the affair and filed for divorce. So the man lost both women, which happens very frequently.

Q. Is there a lesson to convey to men about all of this?

A. An affair won't help a shaky marriage. It almost always makes things worse. So if you *want* to make your marriage work, don't have an affair. Instead, go for professional counseling to resolve your marital or sexual problems. Marriage troubles mostly boil down to a lack of communication and understanding. But once I've started counseling a couple, if one of them has an affair while we're trying to figure out what the problems are in the marriage, it makes the job a hell of a lot more difficult for me and for them.

And in case anyone does not know this truth: There is no perfect mate out there. The ideal lover lives only in your head. Forget about finding her. And face it: *You* are not a perfect mate either. Work on your problems and get smarter about them, because no matter who you're with, there are going to be some problems.

—Russell Segal

Part 6

S E X

20 Ways to Make Love Better

Even if sex is great, perhaps it can be greater.
Read this chapter and you'll be on your way to
becoming an erotic virtuoso.

● ●

FIRST, LET US AFFIRM that we're modern, sensitive guys; we know that having a repertoire of sexual tricks is not the same as sharing love and intimacy. On the other hand, being an erotic virtuoso never hurt love and intimacy one bit. So we've gathered facts and tips that focus on sexual delight for you and your partner. (May she call for encores.) As for intimacy, that angle was already summed up by the classical poet Ovid: "To be loved, be lovable."

1. All work, no foreplay. A hurry-up-and-go lifestyle can lead to speedy ejaculations, warns Sheldon Burman, M.D., director of the Male Sexual Dysfunction Institute in Chicago. "When you have an inordinate amount of stress and not enough time to meet all the demands in your life, your pattern of haste can carry over into the bedroom," Dr. Burman explains. He adds, however, that if premature ejaculation has no physical or deep emotional causes, it often goes away with a lifestyle change, such as reducing stress, quitting smoking, losing weight, and exercising. For more information, call the MSD Institute's 24-hour hotline (except Saturdays) at (312) 725-7722.

2. Try, try again. "I always suggest that people try something new three times," says sex counselor Robert O. Hawkins, Jr., Ph.D., a health sciences professor at the State University of New York at Stony Brook. The first time, he says, you may be worrying about bending your knees and elbows at the proper angle; by the second or third time, you may find you're able to relax and enjoy it.

3. Go buy the book. Sexual handbooks "should be used the way they were intended," says Hawkins. "Sort of like cookbooks, in which you select only the suggestions that suit you."

If your erotic imagination is getting stale, read Nancy Friday's *Men in Love.* Her book describes a wide variety of men's erotic fantasies; it could jump-start your libido.

4. What women wish men knew. Women don't want you to prove your manhood in bed; they want you to have fun. That was some of the good news *Men's Health* heard when conducting a confidential sex survey, asking women "What do you wish men knew about sex?" Other common themes: Don't worry about "The Big O"; women don't care about penis size; slow down, you move too fast; help her tell you what she likes; please discover the *whole* body, guys.

5. When you're hot, you're hot; when you're not, you're not. If you're looking for every sexual encounter to sweep you away on a Technicolor tide of ecstasy, you've been watching too many late-night cable movies. Accept the fact that sex isn't always a fiery welding of souls, advise William Masters, M.D., and Virginia Johnson in their book *Masters and Johnson on Sex and Human Loving.* Sometimes sex is awkward. Sometimes even orgasms are blah. Nobody said men and women had to be sex machines, so relax about your peaks and valleys.

6. The G-spot exists. Some women do have a G-spot, a pleasure area about halfway up the front wall of the vagina, says David M. Quadagno, Ph.D., a medical sciences professor at Florida State University. These women can have intense orgasms from strong, rhythmic pressure against this area inside the vagina. G-spot stimulation in man-on-top positions is heightened by putting a pillow under your partner's hips.

7. Men have hot spots, too. Men have two hot spots that are just waiting for the right touch, says Paul Pearsall, Ph.D., author of *Super Marital Sex.* One area is the small, triangular region on the underside of the head of the penis where a thin strip of skin, the *frenulum,* runs from the head to the shaft. The other area follows the *raphe,* the line you can see and feel that runs lengthwise along the center of the scrotum. Pearsall suggests asking your partner to trace her fingers along this line from behind the scrotum to the front and up the penis.

8. Love potions: real and fake. The prescription form of the drug yohimbine produces erections in about one-quarter of men suffering from impotence, say researchers. (Yocon is the name of the leading prescription yohimbine.) No one knows for sure, but yohimbine, derived from a certain type of African tree bark, may work by boosting blood flow to the penis, by slowing blood flow from it, or by activating pleasure centers in the brain. Whichever, the men for whom it does work get full, sustained erections. Users also report warm spinal shivers, pelvic tingles, and heightened sexual pleasure. Side effects have included increased blood pressure, raised heart rate, and skin flushing.

A word of advice: Just because prescription yohimbine worked for the men in the studies, don't expect to gain sexual powers from over-the-counter or mail-order versions of the drug. The Food and Drug Administration (FDA) has banned the sale of all nonprescription products that claim to arouse or increase sexual desire or improve sexual performance. Among the "aphrodisiacs" the FDA calls useless: ginseng, mandrake, minerals, sarsaparilla, and vitamins.

9. Wake-up sex. Sex in the middle of the night, after you've both had some sleep, can be much more intense, says Michael Morgenstern, author of *How to Make Love to a Woman.*

10. Exercise control. *Kegels* are exercises that give some men stiffer erections and more control over ejaculation by strengthening the muscles of the pelvic floor, say William Hartman, M.D., and Marilyn Fithian, codirectors of the Center for Marital and Sexual Studies in Long Beach, California. Here's the program:

First find the right muscles, the ones you use to stop your urine flow. To exercise them, squeeze them and hold tight. Half your contractions can be brief; hold the rest for 3 seconds. No one will know you're doing Kegels, so you can do them anywhere. Start with a few and work toward 200 a day.

After doing Kegels for a few months, your pelvic muscles will be strong enough to prevent ejaculation if you squeeze them tight just before the urge to ejaculate reaches the "point of no return."

11. The year's best sex. Men have hormonal sex cycles like women's, only subtler. Male sexual potency is maintained by testosterone, secreted by cells in the testicles. The male hormone peaks daily in the early morning and yearly in the fall, according to a study conducted in France. So those cool mornings may be the best time of the year for sex.

• •

Cigs and Babes

Expectant mothers are routinely advised to stop smoking, but fathers-to-be are seldom given the same advice. Some researchers are now recognizing that this may be a serious mistake.

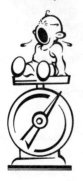

Evidence reported in the British journal *Lancet* suggests that the babies of fathers who smoke only one pack a day average about 5 ounces less at birth and are at greater risk of death than babies of nonsmoking dads—even if the mother doesn't smoke.

This may be a result of the mother and fetus being subjected to passive smoke, but—amazingly enough—some data suggest that the effects may be more fundamental. Cigarette smoke agents have been found in the semen of smokers, implying that risk to the child could go all the way back to conception!

Work in this area is far from conclusive, but a prudent guy ought to consider stopping smoking before he even attempts to conceive a child.

But you don't have to wait until fall to be full of wild oats. Regular exercise makes men feel better about themselves, more relaxed and arousable. In a study of men who began a workout program, more than half said their sex life improved. And the sexual benefits of exercise last. A survey of masters swimmers found that those in their sixties through eighties had sex more than once a week, more typical of 30-year-olds.

Of course, it's possible to overdo a good thing: In one study, male ultramarathoners who ran 100-mile races showed a *decrease* in testosterone.

12. Wham, bam, thank you, sir! Some women get an overwhelming orgasm from quick intercourse without foreplay but with deep penetration, saying it feels different from the orgasms they get from clitoral stimulation or less vigorous intercourse, reports Alex Comfort, M.D., in *More Joy of Sex.* This sort of orgasm produces "gasping, breath holding, and a once-and-for-all climax." Too much foreplay derails this special response, which, when it happens, is as rapid as a man's.

13. Cultivate a sexual appetite. Experts say a low-fat diet may keep you sexually potent as you get older. Tubbing out on foods high in saturated fats and cholesterol may lead to clogged blood vessels, in the penis as well as in the heart, and that can leave you limp. One study showed that clogged penile blood vessels are the main cause of impotence in men over 50.

14. Knowledge is bliss. The basis of great sex is knowledge of your own body and of your partner's: finding out what she likes, letting her know what you like, says Jerome Sherman, Ph.D., a Houston psychologist and president of the 3,000-member American Association of Sex Educators, Counselors, and Therapists. "Then maybe you can enhance the basics with mirrors, colored lights, aromas, lotions, positions, locations—whatever you want to explore," Dr. Sherman says.

15. Some medicines hit below the belt. Some prescription drugs, such as ulcer and blood pressure medicines, can cause temporary impotence. Even over-the-counter drugs like Dramamine (for motion sickness) and Benadryl (for allergies) can have that unpleasant side effect. "Sometimes it takes careful detective work to pinpoint the offending medication, but it is often possible to make substitutions," says Albert McBride, M.D., national spokesperson for the Impotence Foundation (3540 Wilshire Boulevard, Los Angeles, CA 90010).

16. Focus on pleasure, not measure. "I get about four phone calls a week from men who want their penises enlarged or lengthened," says Dr. Sheldon Burman. The average erect human penis is about 5 to 7 inches long, he says, "but guys with normal-sized penises become dismayed because some woman says her last lover was 7½ inches." Although psychological factors may come into play, the mechanism of female orgasm has nothing to do with penis size, says Dr. Burman. "Nine out of ten women have clitoral orgasms, caused by *external* stimulation to the clitoris. If you're physically fit and attractive and an adequate lover, a 4-inch erection is long enough."

For deeper penetration with a short penis, though, Dr. Burman recommends positions "where the woman's thighs won't get in the way." The best: "Woman-on-top, kneeling and facing the man."

17. Soothing the savage breast. Men's breasts have the same potential for erotic pleasure as women's breasts, says Jack Morin, Ph.D., a former health sciences teacher at Skyline College in San Bruno, California. In both sexes, the breasts are richly supplied with nerve endings, especially in the nipple area. Although only half as many men as women get hard nipples spontaneously when aroused, men's nipples are about as likely as women's to become erect when directly stimulated.

18. Keeping score. *Pssst.* Want to buy some sexy software? *Interaction* will provide you with a "personal sexual analysis" based on your answers to 100 multiple-choice questions. An optional module compares your profile with someone else's to let you know if you're compatible. Available for certain IBM, Apple, Atari, Commodore, and Tandy computers, the programs cost $59.95 and $49.95, respectively, or $99.95 for both. Order from IntraCorp, Inc., 14202 Southwest 136th Street, Miami, FL 33186; (800) 468-7226.

19. When once is not enough. Men with low sperm counts can improve their fertility simply by having a second ejaculation 30 to 60 minutes after the first, reports a study in the journal *Fertility and Sterility*. Researchers found that 14 of 20 men who tried the method had higher sperm counts in the second ejaculation, and five of their wives became pregnant. In men with normal sperm counts, however, the second ejaculation usually contains fewer sperm.

20. Silence is wooden. "A lot of my patients complain that their partners don't say anything or are too quiet during lovemaking," says sex therapist Shirley Zussman, Ed.D., co-director of the Association for Male Sexual Dysfunction. "Telling your lover things like 'Oh, you feel so good' and grunting, sighing, making noise—it's all a part of lovemaking," she says. "Good sex is like a light and sound show: Leave the lights on and let out some sound."

—Paul Cooper

Honeymoon Forever

You can keep sex hot between you and your spouse.
These suggestions from top sex therapists
will help you burn down the house.

• • • • • • • • • • • • • • • • • • • •

You worm!

You slug! You vile escargot!

Here you are, happily married or at least happily committed. Maybe you even have kids. And then one day, in an elevator or down a crowded avenue, some protuberant young thing flashes across your line of sight, and in a veritable nanosecond—*a nanosecond, for crying out loud!*—you're ready to make deals with the devil for just 1 hour with her. You're ready to pack it all in. Everything. All the years of marital happiness, the barbecue grill, your joint IRA, the children's future, all of it, just for one lost afternoon. You imagine her thigh seething under her slip as she walks. You imagine things bulging out of their buttons. You imagine exploring every inch of her.

Then she disappears into the crowd and a radiant flush of joy and shame quivers over you. "What kind of a person am I?" you wonder. "And in a friggin' nanosecond!"

Yet the happy fact is that most of the time, we don't act on these impulses. They come and they go, we enjoy them, and we stay married. If the truth be known, most married guys would just as soon stay married. We'd love to keep having hot sex with our wives, and for as long as possible. We'd love to avoid tumbling into some tawdry affair, with all its messy and humiliating consequences. It's not just AIDS and the fact that we're usually too busy or exhausted to attempt the extramarital hunt. It's that deep down, we're basically nice, loving, responsible human beings.

Who would like to get a little more.

So that's the subject of this story—a peculiarly 1990s kind of story, one might say: how nice guys can keep married sex hot for the long haul.

But first, a one-word bit of advice about the whole subject: Relax. There's no reason to doubt your manhood, or your love for your lover, if seeing her naked doesn't arouse you as quickly or as wildly as it once did. It's worrisome, sure. It stirs up all kinds of dark self-doubts. But in a long-term relationship, it's completely natural and predictable to experience a gradual downshift in your sexual responses, and it helps just to know and accept this. You're certainly not alone. (If it's any consolation, there are several hundred thousand other guys reading this story.)

Men's Health rounded up some of the top sex therapists in the country and asked them a very simple question: "How do you keep sex hot—within a marriage?" Following are their suggestions.

VISIT VICTORIA

Okay, sure—sexy lingerie isn't exactly an original idea. But it works. Black lace panties and those little French maid whatchamacallits with the straps have this amazing way of enhancing one's sexual appetite. "It's like she's gift-wrapped," says an 11-year marriage veteran. "And you just want to tear the wrapping off."

One bit of advice: Ask for her size before running to the local lingerie emporium in search of some incendiary undergarment. It's amazing how bad men can be at guessing.

As for choices, if an item turns you on and you give it to her with love, trust that she'll appreciate it. (You might want to take a minute to feel the material before you buy—some of the very slinky stuff can be scratchy.)

SHAKE IT UP

There's a lot of talk nowadays about safe sex, but maybe sex (at least once the protection is in place) isn't supposed to be safe. Maybe it's supposed to be one big, wild, desperate adrenal rush, with stuff getting knocked over and things busting apart at the seams—a few breathless moments stolen from death. Maybe that's why married sex—at least the mechanical kind that we sometimes settle for—often seems hardly worth the trouble. Boredom is death to life and death to sex.

As a result, sex therapists stress the importance of breaking out of boring sexual routines. Alter the pace. Try going much faster, or much slower, than you usually go. And remember, good sex doesn't always have to be lingeringly slow—or terribly considerate. Sometimes she may not mind if you just steal her daisy and run. (In a good relationship, she knows you'll come back later with a bouquet.)

"Try some sessions of nonintercourse sex, where foreplay is the main course, not just an appetizer," suggests Bernie Zilbergeld, Ph.D., a California sex therapist and author of the book *Male Sexuality*. "Or try some sessions where only one person gets all the goodies. Do it one time just for her. Then other times, she'll do it all for you."

If you're always the aggressor, try letting yourself be seduced. And sometimes both can be aggressors. The only limit is your imagination.

● ●

Sex and Fitness

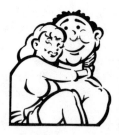

If the promise of better health, a trimmer physique, and a longer life haven't been enough to convince you to exercise regularly, new research pulls out one last ace: The more fit you become as a result of exercise, the more sex you'll have and the better it will be, says a study published in the *Archives of Sexual Behavior*. They're not just talking perceived better. They're talking more orgasms. In the study, 78 healthy but inactive men began exercising aerobically three to five days a week, an hour each day. A control group continued being healthy couch commandos. During the study, each man kept a sexual diary. The results showed that the sex lives of the exercisers significantly improved. The more they exercised, the more and better sex they had. Meanwhile, the sex lives of the nonexercisers were unchanged.

TRY ALL-DAY FOREPLAY

"Always remember that good sex begins while your clothes are still on," say William Masters, M.D., and Virginia Johnson, the granddad and grandma of sex study. "Getting in the mood" is not just the few moments before sex; it can go on for hours, or days, beforehand. Since good sex is just one aspect of a good relationship, it can grow naturally out of the time you spend together.

"The best sex times we ever have usually happen after hours and hours of talking," says one young businessman who's been married five years. "Sometimes, usually it's Saturday, we're talking all day long. The whole day becomes a prelude to bed. If we take the time to reconnect, to really say 'Hello' again, after the madness of the work week, things often get very special after we turn out the lights."

REPOSITION

Address your mate from a new angle. For ideas, take a look at those classic how-to love manuals, *Kama Sutra of Vatsyayana* or *The Perfumed Garden,* an ancient text which describes something in excess of 200 positions. Tell the lady at the bookstore it's for a school paper.

RELOCATE

Sleep specialists tell insomniacs never to read or watch TV or do anything else in bed except sleep. Eventually the bed becomes powerfully associated with the sensation of falling asleep. Beds can also become powerfully associated with boring, predictable sex. So try getting out of the bedroom. "I can't tell you how many people have fantasies of making love in the living room in front of a roaring fire but don't do it," says Dr. Bernie Zilbergeld. "It takes a little effort, but it's worth it. Even if you just do the same old thing, if you try it in a new location, you'd be surprised how much it will add."

Think of yourself as a Hollywood location scout, looking over your whole house for promising stage sets. Consider the kitchen, for instance. Kitchens are full of interesting things. (Remember Jack Nicholson and Jessica Lange on the kitchen table in *The Postman Always Rings Twice?*) Try the walk-in closet. Or the guest bedroom. Or the yard. Or the kids' tree house. Even the car. Just avoid the reflecting pool of the Washington Monument and other extremely public spaces patrolled by park rangers.

RESCHEDULE

Most married couples wind up making love at the same time, every time: After the lights are out and the kids are in bed. But that gets boring, and it probably isn't the greatest time to do it anyway, because both of you are usually exhausted. So try rescheduling the main event. Try the morning—get a babysitter to come Saturday at about 10:00 A.M., then lock the bedroom door and don't come out until you're ready. Try a nooner. Or just skip the late news and go to bed a little earlier.

Some couples are badly in need of synchronized watches. By the time you're ready for bed, she's deep into REM sleep. By the time you're ready to face the day, she's gone. "You're going to have to agree to get up earlier, or go to bed later, in order to spend more working time between the sheets," says one sex therapist.

Therapists often recommend setting aside some time to be together, when you're not stressed out, exhausted, or trying to do two other things at once. (Yes, make a date with her!) Observe Masters and Johnson: "If you don't spend much quality time with your partner outside the bedroom, it's hard to create a sense of closeness and affection the instant you're ready for sex."

Arrange to meet for a drink once a week at 8:30 P.M., after the kids are in bed, just to say hello for 15 minutes. You might be surprised how often these little scenes from a *New Yorker* cartoon turn into scenes from a different sort of magazine.

WARM UP THE VCR

There are certain kinds of videos that can't be watched with a woman without taking a brief, sweet intermission, which may help account for the fact that 20 percent of video rentals now are erotic films. (One company, the Sexuality Library, has begun a home-delivery service for adult videos and books.)

A couple of years ago, a major women's magazine questioned 26,000 of its female readers about their sexual attitudes and proclivities. Eighty-five percent of the women reported having watched at least one sex movie, and almost half reported that they watched them regularly. Said one 26-year-old wife: "My husband and I have had many exciting years of masturbation, oral sex, and intercourse while watching pornographic movies. I feel we have become much closer as a result of our sexual openness."

Dr. Bernie Zilbergeld suggests that if your partner is turned off by hard-core XXX films, you might try something softer. Some experts recommend the films produced by Candida Royale, a former porn star turned producer. (One title: *Every Woman Has a Fantasy*.) Her treatment of explicit action is definitely softer, more feminine, than most XXX fare.

But Dr. Zilbergeld cautions, "You have to remember that you're using erotic films only to increase your arousal; this is not sex education." It's a huge error to judge your own physical endowments, or your sexual performance, against the guys in these films. Most women, confronted by someone like Harry Reems, would call the police. And film editors splice multiple sex acts to make them look like one continuous, marathon performance that, in reality, would kill even the guy in the movie.

ASK, AND YOU'LL PROBABLY RECEIVE

The aforementioned women's magazine survey found that the most sexually satisfied women were the most open with their partner about their sexual fantasies, intimate sexual feelings, and desires. It's safe to conclude that you're much more likely to get what you want if you simply learn to ask for it.

Sounds easy enough, but most of us don't do it. Say Masters and Johnson: "One of the most amazing things to us about sexual behavior is how reticent most people are to talk with their lovers about sex. We see plenty of couples whose well-intentioned caresses fall short of the mark because they're too much, too soon, too little, too light-handed, too far off the mark."

Dr. Bernie Zilbergeld also observes a failure to communicate among the couples he counsels. "Very often, I'll discover that the guy has desires he's never brought up. And the woman says, 'I try to please him, but when I ask him what he wants, he says, "Everything you do is great." ' Women hate that. Men need to learn how to ask."

Don't worry about coming off like a cross between Caligula and the Marquis de Sade. Whatever your fantasy, it's probably not as strange as you think. "Most guys who are reluctant to ask think that what they want is weird or kinky," says Dr. Zilbergeld. "But believe me, there are only so many concave surfaces on the body, and whatever you're thinking of has been tried before."

How to ask? One expert recommends mentally rehearsing your lines before the big moment. (This keeps stuttering, blushing, and mumbling to a minimum.) But maybe you should just relax and do it. "Most women are very open to the idea of trying to make your love life better," says Dr. Zilbergeld. "If you just approach her in a nice, loving way—say, 'I love our sex life, but I'd like for us to try some new ways to keep it interesting'—I think you'd find she may well have some ideas of her own."

That doesn't mean you have to tell her everything. "If you don't feel like sharing, don't," says Dorothy Strauss, Ph.D., a sex therapist and clinical associate professor in the Department of Psychiatry at the State University of New York at Brooklyn. "Sometimes secrets are more delicious staying secrets—unless, of course, they jeopardize your partner's health."

KEEP UP APPEARANCES

"One of the real keys to a satisfying, long-lasting sex life is taking pride in yourself, keeping yourself up," says Dr. Strauss. "Take your physical self seriously; don't let yourself get sloppy." You notice when your mate lets herself go, puts on weight, pads around in her bathrobe all day. It works both ways.

MAKE HER FEEL BEAUTIFUL

One particularly intriguing insight into female sexuality emerged from that women's magazine survey. When asked about the single factor that most inhibited their sexual desires, these women did not report AIDS, pregnancy, guilt, or guys with bad breath. The biggest single sex blocker was insecurity about their own physical appearance. Ashamed of being overweight or not good-looking enough, they found it hard to believe their lovers could be attracted to them.

A word to the wise: Helping your mate feel beautiful is also very likely to make her feel sexier . . . and more willing. Adds Dr. Bernie Zilbergeld: "Very often, the reason that couples have bad sex is that the woman simply doesn't feel attended to. She says, 'He never talks to me, he never pays attention to me, so why should I have sex with him?'"

FOCUS ON THE GAME, NOT THE SCORE

There's something peculiarly male about the idea of focusing single-mindedly on one goal—orgasm—and then driving straight

for it, as though driving to a job. Sex is a form of adult play, a willingness to take time to enjoy things, to go slow *or* fast, to try something
new. Maybe we'd enjoy the game a lot more if we weren't so focused
on the score. And maybe it would last a lot longer.

—Stefan Bechtel

Impotence: Uplifting Solutions

*An expert says your options are many and
your prognosis is good. Here's the scoop on
the latest treatment methods.*

• •

WAITING FOR THE front door to buzz me into the Park Avenue
office of New York City urologist E. Douglas Whitehead, M.D., I get
the feeling the doorman next door is scoping me out, thinking
"Geez, that guy couldn't be more than 34, 35 maybe. Awfully young
to be having trouble getting it up."

I want to explain that I'm just a writer who's come to do a story.
There's nothing the matter with *my* equipment. Luckily, I'm saved
from making a complete fool of myself by the release of the electric
lock.

Minutes later I'm in a warm, comfortable office filled with
framed color prints, where one of the founders of the Association for
Male Sexual Dysfunction has put me at ease talking about a subject
that makes a lot of men, even a lot of doctors, uptight. Soon
hydraulic penile implants cover his desk like so many Datsun spare
parts. He pumps up each model to its maximum hardness and, at
one point, holds a plastic vacuum pump to the crotch of his slacks
and demonstrates it by pumping the device.

Maybe he's not as uninhibited as the British urologist who
capped a lecture at a national meeting of the American Urological
Association on drug treatments for impotence by pulling down his
pants to show off his drug-induced erection ("It happened about
eight years ago and we're still talking about it," Dr. Whitehead says).

But clearly he's no shrinking violet on the subject of sexual medicine.

Were all urologists as down-to-earth and up-to-date as Dr. Whitehead, the world would be a much happier place for the 15 to 20 million American men who suffer from impotence. Unfortunately, only about one-third of the urologists in the United States make impotence and male sexual problems a significant part of their practice.

Dr. Whitehead considers the situation very unfortunate: "At worst, physicians can reflect the same embarrassment that the public often feels in talking about impotence," he says. "Too frequently, I hear about doctors who slap a patient on the back and say, 'Be realistic. You're over 60, you've had enough sex. Just accept it.' But I see patients in their seventies and eighties who are beginning to have trouble getting an erection and *very much* want to do something about it."

If doctors don't talk about impotence, many men won't get help, which is sad. Because according to Dr. Whitehead, 90 percent of cases are treatable, usually without surgery. We asked him to elaborate on the latest developments.

Q. What's new in impotence treatment?
A. The big news of the last ten years is we've discovered that emotional and psychological problems do not cause most cases of impotence. Advances in mapping the blood flow in the penis have shown us that approximately 75 percent of impotence is organic (physically caused).

Q. How can you determine if impotence is actually a psychological problem or a physical one?
A. We interview the patient, using an eight-page questionnaire as a guide. A man usually does not have a physical problem if, for example, he can get an erection during masturbation or sleep or he fails to get erections with one sexual partner but succeeds with another. After the interview, we perform a physical examination, including examining the genitals and looking for signs of excessive female hormones. We also test the pulses to the lower extremities and do a regional neurological exam. Then, if the problem appears to be psychological, we usually refer the patient to a sex therapist or psychiatrist.

● ●

HELP WANTED?

Where to call for information on impotence:

Impotents Anonymous, 2020 Pennsylvania Avenue NW, Suite 292, Washington, DC 20006. Send a self-addressed, stamped envelope for free information. Phone (301) 731-1988 for information about patient support groups around the country.

Impotence Information Center, P.O. Box 9, Minneapolis, MN 55440. Write for the free booklet *Impotence Help in the USA,* or call toll-free, (800) 843-4315.

Impotence Hotline, (800) 558-4321. For general information, pamphlets, and physician listings, write to Surgiteck, 3037 Mount Pleasant Street, Racine, WI 53404.

The phone directory. Dr. E. Douglas Whitehead suggests looking up urologists and selecting one who specifically advertises treatment of sexual impotence, or calling the urology department of a local hospital or medical school for a referral.

● ●

Q. What's the most common physical cause of impotence?
A. The most common one is arteriosclerotic plaque forming on the walls of the penile arteries—a possible consequence of high cholesterol levels in the blood. This narrows the diameter of the vessels that carry blood to the penis. When your body can't deliver enough blood to engorge the penis, it doesn't matter how turned on you are. You will not be able to get or maintain an erection. Sometimes we see other vascular problems, nerve disorders, or hormonal problems, but they're rare.

Q. What kinds of options does a man have?
A. For physical impotence, the available treatments include penile implants, penile injections, vacuum-constriction devices, hormone therapy, and occasionally other forms of surgery. Medicare and other medical insurance policies generally cover treatment costs for organic impotence.

Q. Let's discuss these treatments one at a time. How do penile implants work?
A. There are two general types: noninflatable and inflatable. To understand how they work, you need to picture the anatomy of the

penis: It has two channels within the shaft, one on the left side and one on the right. When not enough blood supplies these channels, or when too much blood drains out, they cannot fill and expand and become rigid. So penile prostheses are implanted, one in each channel, to take over the job of the blood in making the penis erect.

The noninflatable types use a semirigid or bendable rod in each channel, giving you an erection. The rods can be bent by hand. You bend them down close to the body to conceal your penis while dressed; you bend them up into an erection angle to have intercourse. The disadvantages are that there is always a solid shape in the penis you can feel and that the penis doesn't expand in width like it does with the inflatables.

The inflatable implants use two hydraulic cylinders that can be pumped up with fluid. One model is self-contained, with the fluid reservoir and pump combined in the cylinder itself, so the whole system is implanted in the penis. You pump the front tip of the penis several times to inflate an erection. You bend another site downward to drain the penis.

The second kind of inflatable model uses a separate fluid reservoir hidden in the belly and a pump hidden in the scrotum. And the latest models incorporate the reservoir and the pump together in the scrotum. When you're ready to have sex, you feel for the bulb under the skin of the scrotum and press it several times, inflating the cylinders in your penis with fluid. The erection will stay hard for as long as you want, even after ejaculation.

Q. How satisfied are patients with implants?
A. Both types have a success rate of over 90 percent in terms of satisfaction of the patient and his sexual partner. That's the highest success rate of any of the treatments. Another measure of their success is that when there is a malfunction, almost everybody wants the device replaced, not just removed. That, to me, shows they were happy with it.

Q. In the last two devices you mentioned, how natural-seeming is the erection? Would a woman notice anything odd?
A. It appears so natural, a sexual partner might not be able to tell the difference; it can be that good cosmetically. There is only a little scar concealed by the pubic hair, or a little scar on the front of the scrotum, depending on the model and the surgeon's choice of incision.

Q. Is there discomfort for the man with any of these devices?
A. After a week or two or three, most men don't have any discomfort. They say it becomes like part of their body; they don't even think about it being there. Men with implants can have orgasms and ejaculate, and if they are fertile, they can even father children.

Q. The most recent development for impotence is penile injections. How do injections work?
A. There are three types of medication that we use in various combinations and doses: papaverine, phentolamine, and prostaglandin-E1. They all cause the blood vessels to dilate, engorging the penis with blood.

The patient can ask the doctor to determine a dose for an erection that lasts for ½ hour, 1 hour, or 1½ hours, whatever he chooses—but certainly not more than 4 hours. And with the injections, you should not have sex more than eight or ten times a month.

Q. A needle in the penis doesn't exactly sound like it would put you in the mood for sex.
A. The drug is injected at the base of the penis with a very short,

• •

Sperm Like It Cool

The idea of wearing refrigerated underwear to boost fertility is goofy enough for Gene Wilder to don a pair in the comedy *Funny about Love*. But results from the real Testicular Hypothermia Device are no joke. Because too-warm testicles can hinder sperm production, Adrian Zorgniotti, M.D., of the New York University School of Medicine, and engineer Andrew Sealfon invented a gizmo you wear under your clothes as you would a pair of briefs. It keeps the scrotum damp with a trickle of water from a reservoir strapped to your side. The evaporating moisture carries heat away and lowers scrotal temperature by about 2 degrees—enough to significantly improve fertility for men whose sperm is subfertile in count, swimming ability, or shape. Dr. Zorgniotti says that with his device, such men are able to impregnate their mates 53 percent of the time.

tiny-diameter needle. The patient feels a little pinch, if that. The erection usually comes on in 5 to 15 minutes.

Q. What about vacuum devices?

A. You place a suction tube over your penis to draw blood into it, then a constriction ring is slipped off the base of the device onto your penis, trapping the blood inside. After sex you slip off the constriction ring and the erection becomes soft.

Q. What are the disadvantages?

A. For some men the stability is not so good. The ring hardens only the outer two-thirds of the penis, the visible part. So it's a wobbly erection, but usually hard enough for penetration. There can also be a little discomfort, a tightness of the skin, but most patients get used to it. The success rate is 70 to 80 percent, but a lot of men don't want to bother with a vacuum device because it seems so unnatural and cumbersome during foreplay. In my practice, very few patients choose it.

Q. What about hormone therapy?

A. Hormonal problems occur in less than 5 percent of cases. Of those, the most common problem is that the testicles don't produce enough testosterone, the male sex hormone. Occasionally, a problem with another hormone, prolactin, is discovered. I refer all such patients to an endocrinologist. The testosterone-deficient patients receive hormone injections once a month. The outcome is usually successful. The patients with a problem with their prolactin can usually be treated successfully with a medicine called bromocriptine.

Q. Sounds like there are good solutions, yet studies show that more than 60 percent of impotent men put off going to a doctor for a least a year. Many wait five or ten years. What would you say to someone who's begun experiencing problems?

A. There's absolutely no reason to keep impotence a secret, any more than, say, diabetes. The medical profession has to help this process along. Impotence and its treatment is just now starting to be taught at medical schools. And urologists in particular need to help make their patients more comfortable. They, too, are making strides now that effective treatments are available. I think that slowly, the taboo is being lifted.

—Mark Canter

Part 7

DISEASE-FREE LIVING

Can You Catch It?

Not all diseases are created equal. Some are more contagious than others. Knowing whether something is catching is the first step in prevention.

••••••••••••••••••••

SOME GUYS WORRY about catching a cold from the bathroom water glass and cold sores from pay phones. And who knows what microbial assassins lie in wait among those petrified globs of bubble gum stuck to the bottom of the movie seat?

We live among billions and billions of exotic bacteria, viruses, fungal spores, and assorted unseen stuff. Most of these invisible neighbors are harmless, but a few can make you various degrees of sick.

The trick, of course, is to find ways to avoid the harmful bugs and to ignore the others. Doctors are learning more each day about the ways diseases are spread. Here's an updated guide to what you can and can't catch—and how best to protect yourself.

AIDS

We all know by now that AIDS is contagious, but there seems to be a lot of needless concern about getting the disease from casual contact with someone who's infected. The human immunodeficiency virus (HIV) can be transmitted through anal, vaginal, or oral sex with an infected partner or by sharing drug needles with a person who has the virus. That's why those at greatest risk are intravenous drug users and people with numerous sexual partners—homosexuals and heterosexuals alike. "A high level of promiscuity just increases the risk of exposure," says Albert Balows, Ph.D., former assistant director for laboratory sciences at the Centers for Disease Control (CDC) in Atlanta.

Should the paramedic worry about mouth-to-mouth resuscitation? Should the barber toss away his brush and comb? "All we can tell them is to do as they normally would," recommends Dr. Balows. There is no evidence suggesting that AIDS can be transferred through inanimate objects. Small concentrations of the AIDS virus have been found in the saliva of infected people, but former Surgeon General C. Everett Koop, M.D., Sc.D., says that as long as no blood is present, saliva, sweat, and tears pose no threat. "You won't get AIDS from a kiss," he says. Nor from insect bites.

Those who worry about getting AIDS from a blood transfusion should know that the risk of this has been greatly reduced. Blood donors are now screened for risk factors, and donated blood is tested for the AIDS antibody. You cannot become infected when you donate blood.

The surest way to avoid AIDS is to limit sex to one mutually monogamous, uninfected partner. Beyond that, a latex condom, used with a spermicide such as nonoxynol-9, is the best preventive measure.

ATHLETE'S FOOT

Contagious. But for reasons not clearly understood, some people resist the fungus that can cause the itching, burning, and scaling of athlete's foot. Bacteria also play a role in bringing about peeling and blisters.

Athlete's-foot fungi thrive in a moist environment. That's why locker-room shower floors and shoes that don't let the feet breathe can be perfect breeding grounds for athlete's-foot fungi. Topical, over-the-counter antifungal ointments can be effective in banishing the fungi from between toes.

CANKER SORES

Possibly contagious. The cause of these painful mouth ulcers remains a mystery. Experts theorize that they might be spread by kissing or sharing a drinking glass with someone who has a sore.

COMMON COLD

Highly contagious. How does that cold virus find its way from someone else's red nose to yours? Cold viruses attack the upper respiratory tract. When cold sufferers sneeze or cough, they spray extremely fine droplets of virus-bearing mucus and saliva into their environment. "There's no such thing as a dry sneeze," says Dr. Albert Balows. "The smaller the droplets are, the greater the trajectory they have and the longer they float in air."

· ·

Spicy Remedy

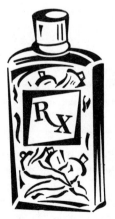

Add hot peppers, curry, and other sizzlers to food when you have a cold: Spices that make your eyes water or your nose run may be modestly effective at clearing up dry coughs. What happens is that when you have a cold, your mucous membranes release less liquid than usual, so the mucus in your lungs and throat gets thick and gummy. Hot, spicy foods "help mucous membranes all over to secrete more liquid, which can help thin mucus," says Varro E. Tyler, Ph.D., professor of pharmacognosy (the study of drugs derived from plants and animals) at Purdue University.

Why do we repeatedly get sick some years? Because there are so many different cold-causing viruses, explains Dr. Balows. "A person can develop a cold from virus number one and, following recovery, may develop an immunity that will protect that person for sometime. But it doesn't give him a nickel's worth of protection from virus number two."

If you don't have a cold, staying away from those who do is the best prevention, although that's easier said than done. In the meantime, the search for a cold cure—a search some researchers consider an impossible dream—goes on. Among the proposed remedies: interferon, a natural antiviral substance produced in the body, now being reproduced in quantity in the laboratory.

DERMATITIS

Contagious. *Pseudomonas aeruginosa* is the full name for the bacterium that flourishes in inadequately chlorinated hot tubs. It causes skin rashes known as "hot-tub dermatitis" as well as swimmer's ear and urinary tract infections. Although such cases are rare, it's also possible to catch pneumonia by inhaling superfine water droplets contaminated with this bacterium. In general, the warm, moist environment of the spa is a disease bug's playground.

ECZEMA

Not contagious. The cause of this itchy skin disease remains unknown, but you can't catch it from someone else. Remedies—not cures—range from topical steroids to cold cloths to diet therapy to a change of climate.

HEPATITIS A

Contagious. The primary mode of transmission is the fecal-oral route—typically when an infected food handler prepares food without first washing his hands. To lessen the likelihood of contracting hepatitis A while dining out, make sure your food is adequately cooked. Washing your own hands frequently reduces the risk of picking up the virus from hand shaking.

HEPATITIS B

Highly contagious. Hepatitis B is usually far more serious—and more common—than hepatitis A. The virus is spread via any exchange of bodily fluids, including blood transfusions, kissing, and anal, oral, or vaginal intercourse. Symptoms usually include joint pain and jaundice, and sufferers are at risk of being afflicted with chronic hepatitis, cirrhosis of the liver, and liver cancer.

HERPES SIMPLEX

Both oral and vaginal herpes can be transmitted through sex—vaginal, oral, or anal—and skin-to-skin contact such as kissing. The virus is most readily (but not exclusively) transmitted when sores are present. In simulated testing, intact latex condoms provided an effective physical barrier against genital herpes during sexual intercourse, but doctors still recommend abstinence when herpes sores are present. That's because the condom only covers the shaft of the penis—sometimes sores can form in other areas of the genital region.

Can you catch herpes from a toilet seat in a public rest room? The odds are extremely low, say the experts. The virus can survive on a plastic toilet seat for about an hour, but for others to contract it, the skin of their thighs or buttocks would probably have to be broken. According to the CDC, there are no documented cases of anyone being infected via a toilet seat. The same goes for public telephones, hot tubs, and swimming pools.

For now at least, there is no cure for herpes. But the prescription drug acyclovir is effective (in pill form) in reducing pain and shortening the period of the virus's activity. (Acyclovir topical ointment is not so effective.) Progress is being made on a vaccine that would prevent herpes infection as well as recurrences in those already infected.

JOCK ITCH

Contagious. Jock itch is caused by the same fungus that causes athlete's foot, so it also thrives under warm, moist conditions. Keeping the infected area dry and using an antifungal topical ointment is usually enough to eradicate the fungus.

STREP THROAT

Contagious. In rare cases, this bacterial infection—characterized by a sore, red throat and high temperature—can lead to rheumatic fever. It's transmitted by direct or by indirect (e.g., sneezing) personal contact. A less-publicized mode of transmission is inadequately refrigerated food. The adaptable bacteria are also known to cause skin infections in athletes who participate in contact sports such as wrestling and rugby.

SYPHILIS

Contagious and still quite prevalent. The disease has four increasingly nasty stages. The first usually consists of painless sores in the genital area and on the lips. The second stage is characterized by a measleslike rash that can cover the entire body. In these stages, syphilis is highly contagious and can be spread via sexual contact, kissing, or any contact with the sores or rash. If syphilis spreads to the eye, it can lead to blindness.

In the third stage, the virus appears to retreat into dormancy, where it can rest for years. Syphilis is not thought to be contagious in this stage. The last stage may not appear for more than 15 years after initial symptoms have disappeared. At this point, the disease is much less contagious, but it can be fatal: The bacteria can invade and damage any part of the body, including the heart, brain, and nervous system.

In the first three stages, syphilis can be cured effectively with antibiotics such as penicillin and tetracycline. In the fourth stage, it may be more resistant to antibiotics and never completely cured. Although a latex condom may provide protection against syphilis if the sores are covered, it's best to abstain from sexual contact if one partner is infected.

TRENCH MOUTH

Not contagious. Although the bacteria that cause trench mouth are thought to be present in many people, only a small percentage of those people suffer with the periodic mouth ulcers and pain. Outbreaks are usually associated with stress or illness.

WARTS

Contagious. You can't catch warts from a frog, but you can get them from another person. Warts are caused by a virus, which enters the skin of the susceptible person through a cut or scratch. Before you can catch warts, your immune system defenses must be lowered, generally through illness. Wart viruses can be picked up either by direct contact or indirectly in moist environments, such as showers or swimming pools.

—Jeff Meade

Shoo the Flu

You don't have to catch the flu this winter!
Catch a bit of good advice and put tissues on hold.

• • • • • • • • • • • • • • • • • • • •

AS A PHARMACIST, I can easily pick out the guy with the flu:
He's the one wandering the aisles, grabbing every cough syrup,
decongestant, pain reliever, and stomach remedy in sight. The
healthier the guy is in general, the more impatient he is with the flu.
He wants a cure and he wants it *now*. Unfortunately, I have to give
him the bad news that there is no cure. His flu bug will continue to
bite until it's good and ready to stop.

The real trick, of course, is for these men to avoid catching the
flu in the first place. A simple trick it isn't: The Centers for Disease
Control (CDC) estimate that in 1990, as many as one person in five
in stricken communities caught the flu. The winter 1989 flu season
was the worst in years, hitting all 50 states; "Influenza was above epidemic levels for ten consecutive weeks, beginning the second week
in January," says Yolanda Mauriz, director of the Flu Track Center.

Over the past ten years, a major flu epidemic has occurred
every year, suggesting that the pattern of epidemics is becoming
more frequent, says Mary Lou Clements, M.D., director of the
Johns Hopkins Center for Immunization Research.

Although there are just three main types of influenza virus
(A, B, and C), they all have unlimited ability to mutate into different
forms. Catching one form will automatically immunize you against
that strain but not against the others.

Usually only one strain of flu predominates during a season,
but instances of two strains circulating at once are being reported.
"Typically an epidemic lasts about six weeks, so when two strains
appear, one after the other, the flu season can be prolonged," says
Dr. Clements.

COUNTERACTING CONTAGION

As any schoolteacher can tell you, it's toughest to avoid the bug
when you're in close contact with people, especially kids. The flu is a
very infectious disease that spreads like wildfire. There may be flu

germs flying around in the air, but the vast majority of them are lurking on people's hands. The more people you touch on a daily basis, the better your chances of getting the flu.

"Both the flu and the common cold are caused by viruses that can be killed by any soap," says Carole Heilman, Ph.D., chief of the Respiratory Diseases Branch at the National Institute of Allergy and Infectious Diseases. If the flu is going around, you'd do well to wash your hands more frequently. When a family member is sick, use a disinfectant spray on the sink, toilet, and tub to kill any lingering germs. You don't have to become another Howard Hughes, but you should keep your distance from people who are sneezing or coughing, even if that means getting off an elevator or changing seats in a theater.

The single most effective way to sidestep the flu is to be vaccinated against it. Like many vaccines, a flu shot actually exposes you to parts of the virus that have been killed and processed in a lab. Your body's immune system identifies and builds antibodies to the virus and is readied for combat if later exposed to a full-fledged viral attack. "The vaccine is 70 to 90 percent effective in preventing flu in people up to age 65," says Walter Gunn, M.D., epidemiologist at the CDC. "And if you do get the flu, the symptoms will be less severe."

Every year, scientists develop a vaccine against the newest strain of the virus. Get your vaccination in late fall or very early winter. Don't wait until the flu's already in town before acting, because the shot takes two weeks to work. Because the vaccine is made using chicken eggs, anyone who is allergic to eggs should not be vaccinated.

• •

Jog with Kleenex

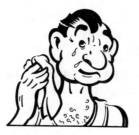

It's usually safe to exercise when you have above-the-neck cold symptoms, such as a runny nose, sneezing, and scratchy throat. But intense workouts are not recommended if you have below-the-neck symptoms, like muscle aches, loss of appetite, a hacking cough, or other upper respiratory ills, or when you have a fever, says the journal *Physician and Sportsmedicine*.

FEELING BETTER

Two relatively new oral drugs—amantadine and rimantadine—can reduce the length and severity of the illness by inhibiting the way the virus reproduces. Both are effective only if given early in the illness—between 24 and 48 hours after the onset of symptoms. They only work against type A influenza, not the B or C strains, but in 1989, A accounted for 99 percent of all flu cases.

If, in spite of all your efforts, you get knocked down by the bug, go home and get in bed for at least the first few days. Drink plenty of fluids. Popping antibiotics like penicillin or tetracycline won't help at all, since antibiotics fight only bacterial, not viral, infections.

Even after the worst of the symptoms is over, you may not feel normal for several weeks. According to research from Nova Scotia, 10 percent of all people with the flu have temporary inflammation of the heart muscle during their fevers. This is one reason why you continue to feel dragged out after your flu has subsided.

Don't be too quick to get back to your exercise program after a bout with the bug; you could be putting extra stress on your heart at a time when it is still recuperating. "If you're used to running 5 or 6 miles a day, don't do it for at least two, possibly four, weeks after the symptoms clear," says Thomas Marrie, M.D., professor of medicine at Dalhousie University in Halifax.

Dr. Marrie and his colleagues warn that subtle yet cumulative cardiac effects are possible, even in people with no history of heart trouble. They also caution against drinking alcoholic beverages during the illness, since alcohol places a strain on the heart muscle. A hot toddy may make you feel better, but skip it and you'll *get* better without hurting your heart.

—Ron Gasbarro

Be Your Body's Best Friend

*How to give the slip to ten common health problems,
including backache, heartburn, and ingrown toenails.*

••••••••••••••••••••

BACKACHE, HEARTBURN, food poisoning, ingrown toenails—
they probably won't kill you, but if you've ever had a bad case, you
won't want to repeat the schooling. Fortunately, doctors and scientists have come up with some pretty good ways to bypass many
everyday health hassles. So learn your lessons the *easy* way. Here's
how to avoid ten common bummers.

ATHLETE'S FOOT

Even if you're an armchair athlete, you're not immune to this
fungus. Athlete's foot is a fungal infection that produces burning
pain, itching, cracked, peeling skin, bleeding, and blisters. Balmy
climates, such as you find inside sweaty shoes, are what makes this
fungus thrive. Once you have it, it takes about four weeks to medi-
cate it away. Here's how not to catch it in the first place.

Don't be a Shoeless Joe. Damp floors can spread athlete's
foot from one health-club member to another. Wear flip-flops in the
locker room, shower room, or spa. After showers, dry your feet
thoroughly. (Use a hair dryer on them if you want, but don't let anyone catch you doing it, or you may never live it down.)

When it's hot, hit the spot. Use Tinactin, Halotex, Desenex,
or another athlete's-foot product daily to weekly in hot weather,
even if you don't have an active case. Spray the insides of your
shoes as well.

Change your shoes. Don't wear the same pair of shoes two
days in a row, advises Chicago podiatrist Dean S. Stern, D.P.M. He
says it takes at least a day for shoes to dry out thoroughly. If your
feet sweat heavily, you may need to change your socks three or four
times a day.

BACK PAIN

Sooner or later, nearly one-half of the guys with blue-collar jobs
and more than one-third of those with desk jobs will end up having

back troubles. These preventive measures can help keep your back younger and trouble-free.

Get up, stand up. "Just stand up for 5 minutes every hour, and I guarantee your back will feel better," says physical therapist Phil Dunphy. "Stand when you talk on the phone, or take a short break to walk around at regular intervals while you're at work."

Or have a seat. Conversely, if your job requires long periods of standing, have a seat every 15 minutes or so, says Suzanne Rodgers, author of *Working with Backache.* The ideal chair, according to the American Medical Association (AMA), has a tiltable back support, adjustable height, and a contoured seat edge that supports three-fourths of your thighs but doesn't cut into the backs of your knees. Adjust the height so you can sit with your feet flat on the floor and your knees level with or slightly higher than your hips. Keep your work surface at elbow height.

Don't read flat writing. Prop your book at a 20-degree angle in front of you, or hold it parallel to your face.

Invest in a good mattress. Hard beds are best and water beds are second best for back pain sufferers because they both evenly distribute weight, according to tests done by the Division of Orthopedics and Rehabilitation at the University of California, San Diego.

Don't offer to help your friends move. Lifting puts more stress on the spine than any other action, especially if it's done wrong. If you must move big stuff, stand close to the object, bend your knees while keeping your back vertical, grasp the object, and hold it as close as you can as you *slowly* stand using your leg muscles. Leaning out and over to lift something, as from the trunk of a car, places an enormous load on your spine and is a notorious slayer of backs. Lay those jumbo bags of dog food on the back seat. Anytime you can use a hand dolly to move heavy objects, do it. Otherwise, push, pull, or slide them.

FOOD POISONING

You get food poisoning two ways: by eating food that actually contains poison, produced by the bacteria growing in it (botulism and staphylococcal food poisoning are this type); or by picking up a bug from food contaminated with organisms (such as salmonella bacteria) that multiply in the body.

Botulism is rare but deadly, killing one-third of the 10 to 15 people who get it each year in the United States. About 75 percent of the cases of botulism are traced to improperly home-canned foods. Here's how to avoid botulism.

When in doubt, toss it out. Scientists estimate that one cupful of the pure botulism toxin could kill all the people on earth. The point is, don't even taste food from a swollen can or from a jar with a swollen lid. Ditto for food that is foamy, moldy, or has a bad odor. Dispose of the food in such a way that there is no chance it will be eaten by street people or by animals.

Unlike botulism, salmonella infection is common: It makes more than five million Americans a year bow to the porcelain goddess. Abdominal pain, diarrhea, and fever are other lowlights of salmonellosis. Avoiding salmonella infection is relatively simple.

Keep your bird cool. Store raw poultry in the refrigerator down low, where it can't drip onto other foods. Rinse it thoroughly before cooking, and dispose of juices from the package. Frozen poultry should be thawed overnight in the refrigerator or in a plastic bag under *cold* water, not just left out.

Don't egg yourself into trouble. Eggs are another potential source of trouble. Skip the Caesar salads and soft-boiled or over-easy eggs. Eggs need to be cooked at least 3 minutes at 140°F to be safe. Use only uncracked eggs and keep them stored no longer than five weeks.

Stow stuff right. Improper storage temperature causes the most cases of food-borne illness, and many occur at picnics. Bear in mind: Bacteria thrive at temperatures between 40° and 150°F. "There is one very simple prevention rule—keep food *hot* or keep it *cold*," says Edmund Zottola, Ph.D., professor of food microbiology at the University of Minnesota.

And cook it well. Unless the inside of your food reaches 165°F or hotter, salmonella could survive. Considering that a study at Iowa State University found salmonella in 41 percent of packaged cut-up chickens, you'd better cook that bird until the inside is white. If you're barbecuing, microwave the pieces for about half the time you would in a microwave recipe, and then throw them on the flames.

Soup cold? Send it back. Restaurants account for about one-half the outbreaks in the United States. Check that the food is well cooked and that hot foods are hot and cold foods are cold. One Food and Drug Administration (FDA) honcho says, "I won't eat warm tuna salad, and I send back soups that are lukewarm."

Sandwich seminar. When you brown-bag it, pack frozen sandwiches, recommends the University of Oklahoma Health Sciences Center. They will thaw by lunchtime. Simple sandwiches freeze best, such as those made with peanut butter, sliced meat, or poultry or with mixtures that do not contain mayonnaise, mayonnaise-type salad dressings, or hard-cooked eggs. Carry lettuce, tomatoes, and dressing to add to sandwiches later.

If possible, keep your sandwich in a refrigerator at work until lunchtime. Some sandwich fillings made with meat, poultry, fish, or egg can spoil if kept at room temperature for more than 2 hours.

HEADACHES

Nine out of ten headaches are caused by muscle tension, according to the National Headache Foundation. Tension headaches usually produce a generalized pain, like a steel band is being tightened around your skull.

Researchers aren't sure what causes the other two types of head pain—migraines and cluster headaches. An estimated five million American men suffer migraines, which typically produce severe, one-sided, throbbing pain, often accompanied by nausea.

While three times as many women suffer migraines, men are cursed with 90 percent of all cluster headaches. Sufferers say these feel like a red-hot poker is trying to get out through the backs of your eyes. These headaches may occur every day for weeks or even months. Men who get them are typically heavy smokers, says Seymour Solomon, M.D., a headache specialist at Montefiore Medical Center in New York.

You're in the best position to recognize what habits and factors bring on your headaches—and perhaps what you can do to prevent them.

Know your danger foods. For some men, it's milk. Others get killer headaches from the monosodium glutamate (MSG) in Chinese food. An amino acid called tyramine, found in nuts, aged cheeses, and chocolate, socks it to others.

Watch the weenies. Pass on the mustard *and* the hot dog. The nitrates in cured meats, including bacon, bologna, and some ham, can dilate blood vessels and bring on major head pain, says Houston's Ninan Mathew, M.D., president of the American Association for the Study of Headache.

Don't sleep through breakfast. Headaches can be brought on by low blood sugar from skipping meals. "A lot of patients get migraines on weekends because they sleep through their normal breakfast time," says Seymour Diamond, M.D., of the Diamond Headache Clinic in Chicago. "It's better to get up, eat, then go back to bed."

Stay loose; sit straight. Working in awkward positions can cause the muscles in your neck to contract and trigger a tension headache, says Dr. Diamond. Check yourself for signs of tightening up—clenched teeth, clenched fists, shoulders up around your ears.

Reach for a rub. Press both thumbs under the bony ridge at the base of the skull where the neck muscles attach. Keep up medium pressure for a few seconds, then release. Don't press too hard, and don't rock or rotate your thumbs. In this way, cover the whole ridge horizontally in a 2-inch-wide band. When you find a hot spot, repeat the thumb-pressure treatment several times.

No strain, no pain. Squinting in the sun or continuous staring at a video display terminal can cause tension headaches. "Take regular breaks from the computer screen and wear sunglasses outdoors," Dr. Diamond advises.

HEARTBURN

Its telltale signs are smoldering pain beneath your breastbone and a sharp, acrid taste in the back of your mouth. The trouble is brought on by a backwash of stomach acid and acid-soaked food sloshing up into the esophagus. A protective lining enables the stomach to withstand its own acid—including the same hydrochloric acid you watched burn a hole in your high-school chemistry lab bench—but the unprotected esophagus becomes inflamed and painful. You usually feel the scorching near the base of your chest, but you could get a burning sensation as high as the back of your throat.

Fortunately, you aren't doomed to continue these slow burns. Doctors know what can cause stomach acid to back up. Change your diet and your ways, and you can extinguish the flames.

Miss the bloat. Overeating is often to blame for getting burned because it puts too much pressure on the esophogeal sphincter, the "door" at the entrance of the stomach. This muscle normally relaxes only to let food *in;* but when your stomach is bloated, the pressure can force food or acid back through it and into your esophagus, says gastroenterologist Frank Moses, M.D., of Walter Reed Army Medical Center in Washington, D.C.

Also, go easy on acidic fruits and vegetables like grapefruits and tomatoes. That goes double for spicy-hot foods—a Gallup Poll found that Mexican cuisine is tops for giving people heartburn, followed by Italian food and pizza.

Don't carbo-load. Carbonated drinks like beer, soda, champagne, and sparkling mineral water can increase stomach pressure, triggering heartburn.

Don't leave the door open to trouble. Avoid cigarettes, alcohol, coffee, chocolate, and sedatives. These can relax the muscle door, leaving it slack enough for stomach lava to erupt into the esophagus.

Don't snack at 10:00 P.M., let alone midnight. If you are prone to heartburn, don't eat anything 2 hours before going to bed. Stomach acid production peaks in the first couple of hours after a meal, and lying down makes you more susceptible to problems.

HEMORRHOIDS

How do you find the hemorrhoid creams at the pharmacy? Head for the aisle full of pained-looking men walking very carefully. Hemorrhoids—swollen, sometimes protruding blood veins of the anus—are a real pain for eight out of ten of us. They're partly hereditary and partly caused by diet and bad bathroom habits. Here's how to avoid the agony.

Go easy. If it's news to you that defecating is not supposed to be a grunting, arduous task, you probably already have hemorrhoids. Straining engorges the veins in the rectum, and hard stools scrape the swollen area, causing more trouble.

Drink fluids, eat fiber. This reduces your chances of constipation and straining on the toilet, says Phoenix rectal surgeon Edmund Leff, M.D.

Lighten up on the salt. Excess salt retains fluids in the circulatory system that can cause bulging of the anal veins.

INGROWN TOENAILS

It seems like a puny problem until you get one. Then it seems like the lightning rod of hell. Here's how to keep on believing it's no big deal.

Avoid pointed or tight shoes. Ingrown toenails occur when a nail—usually on the big toe—grows or is pushed into the soft skin alongside it. Certain shoes will do that. Opt for wide-toed shoes that don't fit too snugly, says Manhattan podiatrist Suzanne Levine, D.P.M.

Don't try shortcuts. Leave your toenails long enough to protect the toe from pressure and friction. To cut them, soften the nails in warm, soapy water, then cut straight across with a sturdy, sharp, straight-edged clipper. Never cut your nails in a rounded shape so that the leading edge curves down into the skin at the sides. Always leave the outside edges of the nail parallel with the skin.

Smooth over your mistakes. If you accidentally cut or break a nail too short, carefully smooth it at the edges with an emery board so that no sharp points are left to dig into the skin.

INSOMNIA

Difficulty falling asleep ranks right behind the common cold, stomach problems, and headaches as a reason why people visit doctors. Here are some commonsense approaches on how to put insomnia to bed.

Stick to a schedule. Try to go to bed and to get up at the same time each day so you can set your system's inner clock, says Merrill Mitler, Ph.D., director of research for the Division of Sleep Medicine at the Scripps Clinic in California. Don't sleep in too late on Saturday and Sunday. If you do, you may have trouble falling asleep Sunday night.

Set aside some quiet time. An hour or so before going to bed, reflect on the day's activities and clear your mind of the distractions and problems that might keep you awake once you pull up the covers, says David Neubauer, M.D., of the Johns Hopkins University Sleep Disorders Center.

Don't turn your bed into a horizontal office. Use your bedroom only for sleep and sex. Don't watch TV, read, argue, talk on the phone, or catch up on paperwork in the sack.

Practice relaxation. Here's an easy technique: Slow down your breathing, and imagine air moving slowly in and out of your body while you breathe from your diaphragm. Do this a few times during the day so it's easy to do before you go to sleep.

MOTION SICKNESS

The water is blue, the boat is white, and you're green from sea-sickness. At first you're afraid you're going to die. After a couple of hours, you're afraid that you're *not* going to.

Motion sickness—be it from a boat, plane, car, or camel ride—occurs when your brain gets confused between motion your inner ears sense and motion your eyes see, explains Horst Konrad, M.D., an ear, nose, and throat specialist at the Southern Illinois University School of Medicine. Once the dizziness, sweating, and nausea begin, motion sickness is as hard to hold back as a cresting wave. Better to steer clear.

Score some Scōp. A prescription drug, Transderm Scōp, comes in a dime-sized patch that you stick behind your ear. It releases sickness-quelling medicine into your skin for up to three days.

Press your luck. The Sea-Band, a woven elastic band worn on each wrist, contains a small plastic button that presses an acupressure point on the inside wrist, which reportedly prevents motion sickness. It's available at some drugstores and marine shops for about $9. For more information, call Sea-Band International at (800) 922-0932.

Go gingerly. Powdered ginger prevents motion sickness better than Dramamine, according to a study at Brigham Young University. You can buy ginger capsules at most health-food stores. Or you can dissolve $\frac{1}{4}$ teaspoon of ginger from your spice rack in hot water or fruit juice and drink it before you travel.

Put up a good front. A cabin in the middle of a large ship does noticeably less rolling and pitching. In a car or bus, sit up front and focus on the road ahead as if you were driving. If you must read, slouch down in the seat and hold the reading material close to eye level to block out your side vision of the scenery rushing by.

TRAVELER'S DIARRHEA

Also known by a slew of ethnic slurs, it's caused by foreign strains of bacteria that normally live in your intestines and aid with digestion. These strains give you diarrhea by producing a toxin that prevents your bowels from absorbing water from fluids and foods—extra water that has to come out somehow. Okay, no more. Here's how to give it a wide berth.

Don't try everything on the menu. Avoid uncooked vegetables and fruits you can't peel, undercooked meat, raw shellfish, ice cubes, and cocktails mixed with anything but bottled water (contrary to popular belief, the alcohol won't kill the bug).

Turn off the tap. When possible, stick to bottled water for drinking. Boiling water for 3 to 5 minutes purifies it, as do iodine droplets or tablets. (You can buy these at most camping stores. Follow the instructions.)

Drink orange juice or colas. Acidic liquids can help keep down the bacteria count in your gut.

Buy some trip therapy. Drink lots of acidophilus milk and eat yogurt. These foods provide a healthy level of beneficial bacteria in your colon that can help ward off a bacterial invasion. (Frozen yogurt may not work, since much of it contains no active yogurt culture.) You can buy capsules containing acidophilus and take them during the trip.

—Richard Stevens

Farewell to Knee Pain

Treat your knees right, and they'll carry you the distance. Here's how to get a leg up on the most common of problems.

• •

IT'S NOT REALLY FAIR the way knee injuries occur. Take the case of Gerry, an engineer in his forties, whose knee started acting up after a minor ski accident. (A less experienced skier rammed him from behind—while he was getting off the lift, no less.) Gerry's no sofa pilot. He keeps in shape, and he's devoted to a number of outdoor sports. His doctor had him in a leg immobilizer for a while, then put him on a regimen of leg-strengthening exercises. Pretty soon—too soon—Gerry was back to one of his favorite sports: speedwalking. His rehab, however, had built up only some of the muscles in his injured leg, and that caused an imbalance. The result was a classic case of runner's knee.

Whether we're young, old, or middle-aged, the knee is our most vulnerable joint. It's also a repeat offender: Once you've seriously injured a knee, your odds of reinjuring it are astronomical. But you can beat those odds if you practice a little prevention and get prompt medical attention at the first sign of trouble.

Why is the knee such a sore spot? Partly because it's not one of nature's best engineering jobs. "The knee is essentially a ball sitting on a flat surface, held in place by four rubber bands," says James Fox, M.D., an orthopedic surgeon and author of the book *Save Your Knees*. "It's a perfectly good joint—for an animal that lived millions of years ago and walked on all fours."

Those of us who live today and walk on two legs tend to put a lot of stress and strain on our knees. We gain weight. We try to lose it by jogging, skiing, playing football and basketball. We get a little pain, but we write it off to being "out of shape." Even worse, we try to work through the discomfort. The words of Little League and junior-varsity coaches from our past egg us on: "Whatsa matter, *(your name here)?* Gonna let a little *pain* slow you down? My grandmother can move faster than that, and she uses a walker!"

But "no pain, no gain" is the *wrong* philosophy, especially when dealing with knees. Pain in the joint itself indicates a problem that can only get worse if not treated. Fortunately, in nine out of ten cases, knee problems can be treated rather conservatively, with immediate rest and subsequent physical therapy. In cases where a knee injury does require surgery, a thin, tubelike instrument called an arthroscope makes it possible to do complex repairs through a few small holes in the skin, greatly reducing recovery time.

Gerry took his knee to Elliott B. Hershman, M.D., an orthopedic surgeon at the Nicholas Institute of Sports Medicine at Lenox Hill Hospital in New York City. Dr. Hershman prescribed hip-abductor exercises to strengthen the quadriceps. "By bending at the hip instead of the knee, he worked the muscles without aggravating the injured joint," Dr. Hershman explains. How does Gerry feel now? "Great! A year after the injury I was back on the slopes," he says. And for an active man, that is the true test of any cure.

GET A LEG UP ON THE PROBLEM

The kneecap, or patella, is the focus of the most common kind of knee pain: *chondromalacia patella.* It's often called runner's knee, but it strikes nonrunners as well—as Gerry could tell you.

Runner's knee can feel like a generalized, dull ache in the front of the knee or a very specific, sharp pain of the inner surface of the kneecap. The pain is caused by damage to the cartilage behind the kneecap. "The first stage is a softening of the cartilage, but eventually it gets chewed up," says Lyle L. Micheli, M.D., president of the American College of Sports Medicine and associate professor of orthopedics at Harvard University. "It's the result of excess or uneven pressure on the kneecap during activity."

If you have runner's knee, it's of primary importance to stop aggravating the injury. "The first thing I get my patients to do is cut back to a comfortable level of activity," says James G. Garrick, M.D., an orthopedic surgeon and director of the Center for Sports Medicine at St. Francis Memorial Hospital in San Francisco.

When the knee stops hurting, that's half the battle. The other half is for your doctor to figure out exactly how the knee got hurt. Three frequently interrelated problems cause runner's knee.

1. Overtraining or starting a new workout: Trying to do too much too soon can wreak havoc on more than your knees.

2. Hidden weaknesses: Sometimes one of the four muscles that make up the quadriceps isn't pulling its own weight. Often this is the *vastus medialis,* which keeps the kneecap on the right track as it moves up and down. It's also possible for the hamstrings (rear thigh muscles) and calf muscles to be too tight in relation to the quadriceps.

3. Structural flaws: Barely noticeable misalignments of the leg and foot cause the kneecap not to move properly in its groove. These can be problems you're born with, like being knock-kneed or pigeon-toed, or they can be brought on by external factors, such as too much running on an uneven surface.

While strengthening—usually starting with gentle-on-the-joints isometric exercises and graduating to light weight lifting—can correct training errors and muscle imbalances, it can't help all cases of misalignment. Sometimes prescription orthotic insoles are required.

More aggressive tactics include putting the patient on crutches for a few weeks and, rarely, giving injections of anti-inflammatory drugs. Surgery is a last resort.

One procedure for misalignment problems involves partially severing some of the tendons that attach to the outer edge of the kneecap. This allows the quadriceps to pull the kneecap inward and back into line. The other surgical option is to smooth down the cartilage surfaces on the front of the thigh bone and behind the kneecap through arthroscopic surgery.

The next most common knee injury is a cartilage tear, although perhaps that's a misleading term. "It's not surface cartilage that tears, but two movable cartilage shock absorbers in the knee called *menisci*," explains Robert Bielen, M.D., a sports medicine specialist and clinical assistant professor at the University of California, Irvine.

A tear is often caused by a specific accident. Sam, a hotel manager in his fifties, had just crossed the finish line of a Central Park road race when another runner rammed into him. "He was showing off for the TV cameras. I landed on my knees and heard a pop. The medics cleaned out the scrapes and told me I'd be fine. But over the next few months, I noticed the knee bothered me whenever I ran," he remembers.

Symptoms of a meniscal tear are sharp pain at the joint line when you move and slipping or locking of the joint. Tears generally don't heal on their own—especially tears toward the meniscus center, where blood supply is poor. "But there's good evidence that a tear on the edge of the meniscus will heal, especially if it's stitched up," says Dr. Micheli. When the tear is in the middle of the meniscus, surgeons just try to smooth out the rough spots. The most common way is to shave down the ragged edges of the tear with tiny instruments manipulated through an arthroscope. Another approach is to zap the edges of the tear with a laser, a relatively uncommon but effective procedure.

Sam, who, like Gerry, was a patient of Dr. Elliott Hershman, was advised to have surgery, since the tear was on the edge of the meniscus. "It was a flap tear that wouldn't compromise the shock-absorbing qualities of the meniscus, so I removed the torn flap," Dr. Hershman explains. Sam is back to running every day: "A year later, and I can't even find the scars!"

TEARS THAT BRING TEARS

Torn ligaments are also responsible for knee pain. Of the four ligaments that stabilize the knee, the one most likely to stretch or snap is the anterior cruciate ligament, or ACL.

• •

TWIN PEAKS: PUMPING UP YOUR KNEES

The best way to prevent a knee injury is to keep the muscles that operate the knees in peak condition. That's what these exercises are
designed to do. Just be sure to get your doctor's okay first, as some of
these exercises could aggravate preexisting injuries, especially if done
too soon or with too much weight.

You can do most of these exercises on the kind of weight machines found at a gym, or you can buy ankle weights for home use.
Two inexpensive alternatives: penny rolls (about three to a pound) and
lead fishing sinkers. Put them in a sock, knot the end securely, and
drape the sock over your ankle. When you work up to more weight,
you can put your pennies in a runner's fanny pack and hang the strap
over your ankle.

If any of these exercises hurt, stop immediately. Try less weight
or no weight. You want to feel muscle burn, but pain anywhere in the
joint is a signal to back off.

1. Straight-leg raise. Lie on your back on a hard surface. Bend
one leg at the knee, keeping the foot flat on the floor. Lock the knee of
the other leg in an extended position and lift from the hip. Raise your
foot no more than 6 or 8 inches and hold for about 6 seconds. Then
drop your leg and rest for 6 seconds. Do ten repetitions of this exer-

• •

The ACL stabilizes the knee from front to back—the direction
in which you're most likely to overstress it. The ACL keeps the tibia
(shin bone) from sliding forward and out from under the femur.

Ligaments can stretch about 6 percent of their length. After
that, they snap. "You can have a partial tear of the ACL," says Dr.
Lyle Micheli, "but most are clean breaks." This injury usually occurs
during sudden stops and twists in football or soccer or when jumping and landing in basketball or volleyball. If you pull one of these
moves and hear a loud pop, chances are you've snapped the ACL.
Swelling follows.

"I didn't hear a pop, but I had only a partial tear of the ligament—at first," says Andrew, a lawyer in his late twenties. He was
playing a friendly game of basketball when he twisted the wrong

• •

cise with your right leg, then ten with your left.

You may want to start without weights. Gradually add weight as you gain strength—up to about 5 pounds maximum. Then, rather than adding weight, see if you can hold your leg up for 10 seconds instead of 6 without shaking. You can eventually build up to three sets of ten repetitions.

2. Seated quadriceps extensions. Sit in a chair with your legs bent at the knee and hanging down. With a comfortable amount of ankle weight, raise your legs two-thirds of the way and hold for 6 seconds, then rest. Repeat ten times. Don't extend your legs straight out, because the extra stress will do more harm than good. Gym version: This exercise can be duplicated at the gym on a thigh-and-knee weight machine.

3. Hamstring strengthener. Stand facing a wall, with your hands braced against it for stability. With your ankle weight secured, lift your foot and slowly bring your shin to a 90-degree angle with the floor. Hold for 6 seconds, then slowly lower your foot. Do ten repetitions with each foot. This exercise can be duplicated on a thigh-and-knee weight machine. The only difference is that you lie on your stomach, pulling the weight until your feet are pointing straight up.

• •

way during an attempted hot-shot move. "I fell facedown in horrible pain. It was so bad I had difficulty breathing," he recalls. "My first reaction was to try to walk it off, but it quickly became apparent I needed to go to a doctor."

Most ACL tears are diagnosed by a physical exam and the patient's description of what happened. Two high-tech methods can be used to confirm the diagnosis: arthroscopic examination and magnetic resonance imaging (MRI). (Ligaments don't show up clearly on x-rays.) Andrew underwent an MRI and was told his ligament was severed. But then a closer look through an arthroscope showed that he actually had 30 percent of the ligament left intact. If the blood flow to the ACL wasn't disrupted, there would be a chance of saving it.

Surgery isn't required in every instance of an ACL tear or break, but not fixing the damage will limit a person's mobility somewhat. Simple exercises to strengthen the muscles around the knee can give adequate stability for most everyday activities. "The first doctor I went to told me to learn to love biking and golfing," says Andrew. You can also walk, run, and swim with a severed ACL. But climbing, carrying heavy objects, or walking on uneven ground is difficult.

Andrew eventually had to undergo ligament-replacement surgery when his ACL deteriorated because of poor blood flow. There are three types of replacement ligaments, listed here in order of preference:

■ A transplant from the patient's own body, using part of either a leg tendon or hamstring

■ A part-natural, part-synthetic transplant called a *stent*, in which a tiny piece of polypropylene rope strengthens a replacement tendon

■ A completely artificial tendon made of Gore-Tex (yes, it's the same thing they make raincoats from)

Andrew's doctor, Ralph A. Gambardella, M.D., an orthopedic surgeon at the Kerlan-Jobe Orthopedic Clinic in Inglewood, California, chose to transplant a piece of Andrew's own patellar tendon, which runs from the kneecap to the shin. In general, the success rate with ligament-replacement surgery is 90 percent or better, but the road to full recovery is long and requires sticking to a strict physical-therapy regimen.

"My knee will never be exactly the same, but I've come a lot farther after a few months of rehab than I ever expected," Andrew says. "After the injury, I swore I'd never set foot on a basketball court again. Now, Dr. Gambardella actually encourages me to play slow-motion one-on-one as part of my therapy. My hook-shot days might not be over just yet."

—*Steven Lally*

How to Spot an Ulcer

*Only 25 percent of men who think they have ulcers
really do. Let Dr. Michael Oppenheim
put your worries to rest.*

• • • • • • • • • • • • • • • • • • • •

IF YOU HAVE BIG-LEAGUE acid pain on an empty stomach or at least 2 hours after a meal, it's okay to worry about an ulcer. Your doctor will also worry, because that matches the classic ulcer description from medical books.

Although my patients and I worry a great deal about ulcers, we're usually wrong. Only about 25 percent of patients with typical ulcer symptoms actually have ulcers. Most of the rest have something called *nonulcer dyspepsia,* which basically means that diagnostic tests find nothing wrong. Many of the others have *gastritis,* a vague term applied to empty-stomach pain.

When a patient comes to me with empty-stomach pain, I ask the following questions. You can do the same at home.

Does food or antacid help? Ulcers hurt most when stomach acid irritates them. Food and antacids help dissipate the acid, diminishing the pain. So if food or antacids help eliminate the pain, it hints at an ulcer. Unfortunately, food and antacids also help eliminate the pain of gastritis and nonulcer dyspepsia, so you can't hang a diagnosis on this answer alone.

Does any food aggravate the pain? Most patients tell me fruit juice and spicy food make their pain worse. I solemnly advise them to avoid these things in the future (sometimes practicing medicine is easy). However, food intolerance is so common, it's not exactly a diagnostic thunderbolt.

What other symptoms do you have? Victims of nonulcer dyspepsia often complain of bloating, belching, nausea, heartburn, and a feeling of fullness. Occasionally they vomit. These symptoms occur less often in ulcer cases but often enough to make them unreliable clues.

Does aspirin upset your stomach? About two-thirds of ulcer patients have this problem, so it's pretty good evidence.

Do you have pain at night? Stomach-acid secretion peaks

around 2:00 A.M., so symptoms that wake you up long before dawn should open your doctor's eyes. On the other hand, nocturnal pain occurs in every stomach disease and with ulcerlike frequency in nonulcer dyspepsia.

Okay, so these are pretty feeble clues on which to base an ulcer diagnosis. Here are the only scientifically proven risk factors for ulcers in someone with empty-stomach pain:

- Being male
- Being over 50
- Smoking
- Having had an ulcer in the past

Isn't science wonderful? The first three items are risk factors for almost any disease you can think of. And the fourth merely restates the medical cliché "Once an ulcer, always an ulcer" (in other words, most ulcers recur).

So can you tell whether you have an ulcer without medical tests? You already know part of the answer: *You can't.* Here's the rest: *It doesn't matter.*

The reason is that my treatment is the same for ulcers, gastritis, and nonulcer dyspepsia. If you come to my office with garden-variety empty-stomach pain, I'll ask the questions above, then give the treatment below. I don't order tests unless this treatment fails. To most people, this approach wouldn't classify me as a particularly sensible and economical doctor, although that's what I am. It's good medical practice.

You can treat yourself at home by doing the following things.

Eliminate stomach irritants, especially smoking. I allow up to two cups of coffee a day, provided they don't obviously aggravate pain.

Prevent pain by suppressing acid. Take 2 tablespoons of over-the-counter liquid antacid 1 hour and 3 hours after meals and again at bedtime. Don't worry that the label advises far less. Antacid labels always recommend too little. Antacids are safe; the only common complications of high doses are diarrhea or constipation. If you suffer from these unwanted side effects, try different brands.

Home treatment does have its limits. If seven days of this therapy give no relief at all, see a doctor. But if this treatment works, you should be pain-free in a month.

—Michael Oppenheim, M.D.

It's All in the Wrist

Don't get stuck in the carpal tunnel syndrome.
Carpenters, musicians, gardeners, computer
users, and all you other guys who use your
hands a lot—read this!

● ●

IN SIMPLER TIMES, "a flick of the wrist" meant something easy
and harmless. But no more. In this high-tech era of computer keyboards, power tools, and increased demands for productivity, a flick
of the wrist can become the source of burning pain, tingling fingers,
numbness and weakness in the hands, and, at its worst, permanent
neurological damage and short-circuited careers.

Scott Fleming's symptoms struck at night. His forearms would
cramp, and his hands would curl into tight claws. "My wife would
wake me up and tell me, 'You're groaning again,' " the 41-year-old
former carpenter recalls. "I could swing a hammer all day, but if I
had to drive screws, my hands would get really tired."

John G. Taylor's problems began with a pain in his right wrist,
arm, and shoulder and tingling in the tips of his fingers. The symptoms have since spread to his left wrist. A journalist, Taylor, 40, is
finding it increasingly difficult to type. "I've been in this business for
23 years," he says. "It's devastating to think I might have to find
something else to do, but I've exhausted almost all my options. I
may not have a choice."

UNDER THE SURFACE

The source of all this misery: carpal tunnel syndrome (CTS), a
compression of the wrist's median nerve, which gives movement
and sensation to the thumb and first three fingers. In one of nature's
rare traffic jams, nine tendons, an artery, and a vein shoot out of the
comparatively spacious forearm and join the median nerve to con-
verge on the carpal tunnel—a narrow passageway through the
bones of the wrist—before passing into the hand. Even under the
best of circumstances, it's a snug fit.

"When you move your fingers, the tendons slide back and
forth inside the tunnel," explains David Thompson, Ph.D., an

ergonomist in the Industrial Engineering Department at Stanford University. "If you bend the wrist and then move the fingers, the tendons pull through at an angle, rubbing against each other."

Too much of that kind of friction irritates the tendons, making them swell. And with no room to expand inside the tunnel, the swollen tendons press on the median nerve. "It's like stepping on a hose with water coming out," Dr. Thompson explains. "The nerve impulses are slowed down, and some might not be able to get through at all. You lose sensation in the fingers; they don't work right."

CTS is a disease of the times, a clash between anatomy and labor-saving technologies that require less sweat but more repetitive handwork. It hits carpenters, musicians, butchers and meat packers, auto workers, gardeners, construction workers, supermarket checkers, assembly-line workers, writers using computer keyboards—anyone who uses his hands repetitively with the wrists bent.

By some estimates, one in ten Americans will get it. Women used to get CTS more than men, but that's changing. "In my practice, it's now about evenly divided between men and women," says Allan Bernstein, M.D., a neurologist in Hayward, California. The reason: More men are moving away from heavy manual labor into tasks requiring repetitive hand motions.

John Taylor blames his case on word processors. Computers were hailed as timesavers for writers and editors: No more stopping to change ribbons, to put in a new sheet of paper, to unstick recalcitrant keys. But those temperamental old manuals were actually easier on the wrists. "The old typewriters would go only so fast. Every few seconds, you'd have to stop and return the carriage or press the carriage return or put in a new sheet of paper," explains Linda Frisbey, a physical therapist in Berkeley, California. "Those brief pauses were enough to give the wrists a rest."

CAUSES AND CURES

Not all CTS is job-related, however. John Mello, 40, a guitar maker, began having problems when he took some time off from work to do some wiring and plastering in his house. "After two weeks of snipping 12-gauge wire and holding trowels, I started waking up at night with numb hands and an incredible ache up and down my arms," he says.

• •

DON'T THROW YOUR WRIST A CURVEBALL

Certain kinds of work have been tagged as the primary cause of carpal tunnel syndrome. Now it seems some forms of play may aggravate the condition. CTS can be made worse by sports that strain the wrists, says Susan Toth Cohen, an occupational therapist and assistant clinical professor at Thomas Jefferson University in Philadelphia. If you're already at risk on the job, protect yourself during these activities.

Weight lifting. If you wrap your wrists too tightly, the straps can cause swelling and make your hands stiff. "But as a reminder to keep your wrists straight," Toth Cohen says, "the straps are great."

Running. Avoid clenching or squeezing your hands while running. Hand weights may also aggravate the condition.

Exercise machines. On stair climbers, avoid leaning on the handrails during increased speeds, which places the wrist in an unnatural position. The continuous flexing and extending of the wrist on stationary bicycles and rowers can aggravate CTS symptoms.

Racquet sports. Gripping the racquet correctly and keeping aware of wrist position is the best defense against CTS. If you do develop symptoms of CTS while playing racquetball, squash, or tennis, you may be wise to find another sport. But don't assume that if you have pain or tingling in your hand or wrists, you have CTS. See your doctor.

• •

Nighttime hand pain or numbness is a classic CTS symptom. "People retain more fluid at night, which increases pressure on the median nerve," explains Dr. Allan Bernstein. Other symptoms include a burning sensation in the first three fingers and tingling and numbness. Sometimes the pain strikes higher up the arm, and for reasons not clearly understood, CTS can even cause pain in the neck, often confusing the diagnosis.

At its severest, the syndrome can permanently damage the median nerve. This results in loss of sensitivity and weakness, making it increasingly difficult to hold and control even the lightest objects.

"The hand is a remarkable structure, literally an extension of the brain," says James Stark, M.D., a San Francisco specialist in physical rehabilitation. "Your hands are another pair of eyes when you can't see; the sensory feedback that comes back along the median nerve is very important in our lives. When the nerve is damaged and sensation is lost, it's almost like you've lost your ability to see in the dark."

If you think you have symptoms, first see a doctor to rule out other possible causes. If CTS is diagnosed, healing may require a week or two of rest, perhaps with the wrist in a splint. Hot soaks and an anti-inflammatory drug like aspirin can also help. In severe cases, steroids are injected into the carpal tunnel to reduce swelling.

Dr. Bernstein thinks CTS may be linked to a B-vitamin deficiency that causes swelling on the nerves and a lowered pain threshold. He prescribes B_6 in initial daily oral doses of 150 milligrams (about 75 times the Recommended Dietary Allowance), reducing that dosage to 25 milligrams over six months. However, he cautions that this therapy should be undertaken only with a doctor's supervision, as high doses of B_6 can be toxic.

WHEN THE GOING GETS TOUGH

Surgery, the last resort, is performed when conservative therapy fails. It's an outpatient procedure done under local anesthetic. An incision is made in the palm to expose the ligament covering the top of the carpal tunnel. Then the ligament is cut. "The ends literally snap apart," says John Sebright, M.D., assistant clinical professor of surgery at Michigan State University. "That allows the tunnel to spread, providing more room inside for the tendons, blood vessels, and the median nerve." Scar tissue fills in the gaps, essentially making the ligament longer. The cost is $1,500 to $2,000 a wrist. You're in a splint for a week or two, although total recovery may take longer.

Scott Fleming, the carpenter, had surgery on both wrists about six months after his night pain started. A week later he was back on the job, and he felt completely recovered in about a month. "I haven't experienced any change in my grip or grip strength," Fleming notes. "I lift weights and everything's fine."

Another procedure, also performed under a local anesthetic, requires a ½-inch incision in the crease in the wrist. In this operation, the surgeon can't ensure that the ligament he's cutting is the cause of the pain, although a preoperative lab test called an *electromyogram* may confirm a diagnosis of CTS. According to

David M. Pagnanelli, M.D., assistant professor of neurosurgery at the Medical College of Pennsylvania, "The technique requires no postoperative splinting of the wrist and no physical therapy to restore the wrist to optimal physical functioning." The cost: about $1,500.

But neither kind of surgery cures all cases. Notes Roger Stephens, Ph.D., a government ergonomist: "In my experience, about only one in four patients with true, work-induced CTS can return to the job successfully. We're seeing many job changes."

MOUNTING AN OFFENSIVE

Obviously, it's a much better idea to prevent CTS in the first place. The key is body mechanics. "Sometimes changing the height of your chair or the way you hold a tool can cure the problem," Dr. Stephens says. Here are some things you can do:

■ Type with your arms parallel to the floor and your wrists in neutral, "floating" above the keyboard. Adjust the height of your keyboard, desk top, or chair to eliminate any cocking of the hands. Don't rest your wrists on the edge of the desk. That puts compression on the carpal area.

■ If you have a detachable keyboard with a long cord, change your position occasionally. For instance, rest the keyboard on your lap. Consider a wrist rest, a soft pad that extends toward you from under the keyboard. Ergonomic Design Inc. (303-452-8006) sells one for about $50. Sit-Rite (800-235-4204) markets an adjustable rest for about $350.

■ Switch from a conventional computer mouse to a track ball, which looks like a pool ball resting in a cup. "We see more and more engineers and designers getting CTS," says David Rempel, M.D., an ergonomist at the University of California, San Francisco, and an expert in occupational medicine. One reason is that clicking and dragging a mouse is tough on tendons. A track ball is easier to lock and release.

■ Use larger tool handles. "Too small, and they can press directly on the tendons and median nerve in the palm," explains Dr. Rempel. Buy soft covers that enlarge tool handles, or make your own with duct tape and foam rubber.

■ Avoid working in the cold, when tendons are less flexible and more likely to become irritated and swollen.

■ Avoid repetition. "Take a break lasting 5 to 10 minutes every hour and shorter pauses every 5 to 10 minutes," advises Dr. David Thompson. "Shake out your hands, roll your head on your shoulders, get up and walk around—anything to relax and get the blood flowing."

John Taylor's newspaper has spent hundreds of thousands of dollars on adjustable desks and chairs, computers that automatically remind the user to take a break, and other work aids to prevent repetitive-strain injuries like CTS. "Those changes have reduced the incidence among those who didn't already have CTS," Taylor says. But he wonders whether it might be too late for him. Conservative measures have so far failed. He's considering surgery and, if that doesn't do it, the grim prospect of a job change at the height of his career.

John Mello's symptoms cleared up as soon as he finished his plastering. "But I think I'm sensitized," he says. "I did a little touch-up one day, and that night, the pain was almost as bad as it was at its worst. I'm lucky, though; my work is hand-intensive, but it doesn't aggravate the problem."

Scott Fleming became a project supervisor not long after recovering from wrist surgery. Whether because of the surgery or the job change, he hasn't had any problems since.

—Eric Olsen

Now Hear This ...

A bit of caution can save your ears. Hearing specialists tell you how to protect an invaluable sense.

• • • • • • • • • • • • • • • • • • • •

ROD STEWART, PETE Townshend, and Ted Nugent may not have all that much in common musically, but they do share one thing: None of them can hear a pin drop . . . or a pen, for that matter. Years of screeching feedback, howling riffs, and exploding smoke bombs have left each of them with permanent hearing damage.

"I gave up my electric guitar decades ago," you say; "What's this got to do with me?" Well, for one thing, it's not just the guys *playing* the music who get their ears blown off.

"If checked immediately after a rock concert, many people will show a temporary reduction in hearing," says ear specialist James Donaldson, M.D., of the University of Washington School of Medicine. "If it doesn't get better within 12 or 16 hours, the loss is usually permanent."

Nor is it only rock music that can shake, rattle, and wreck your hearing. Chronic exposure to much lower decibel noises can, over time, lead to serious problems.

EARS ARE GOOD FOR YEARS

Doctors once believed that declining hearing was a normal part of aging. After all, one out of two men over the age of 65 has hearing loss serious enough to interfere with normal conversation. But when scientists tested older people in more primitive societies, they found little or no hearing loss. The passing years don't ruin your ears, in other words; the passing sirens and the passing boom boxes do.

Deafness caused by loud noise in its many forms accounts for more than one-third of the total cases of hearing loss in the United States. Experts say men are most at risk. "Men tend to live noisier lives," says Dr. Donaldson. "They're exposed to more noise in both their work and play."

Modern medicine can do lots of impressive things, but one thing it can't do is bring back your hearing from the dead. No medication or surgery can provide a cure for noise-caused hearing loss. "You treat it by wearing a hearing aid or learning to read lips," Dr. Donaldson says.

Call it another form of hair loss. Inside your ears are tiny, hair-like nerve cells, called cilia, that convert vibrations into electric signals that are sent to the brain, where hearing actually takes place. A relentless racket can flatten the cilia, dampening hearing until the cells regain their upright position. That may take hours. Repeated bombardments can kill the delicate cells. As cilia die, hearing is impaired, never to return to normal. The harm done depends on the volume and on how long your ears drown in the sound. "Anything that's loud enough to interfere with normal conversation between two people at arm's length is loud enough to damage hearing if you listen to it regularly," Dr. Donaldson says.

NOISES THAT DEAFEN

In general, noise that is 85 decibels or louder is potentially harmful. (Busy traffic averages about 75 to 85 decibels, a lawn mower about 90.) Chronic exposure to noise 85 decibels and louder can, over time, irreversibly damage hearing. As the din rises, so does the danger: A chain saw (100 decibels) or a rock concert (115 decibels) can injure your hearing in as little as 2 hours.

There may not even be any warning that something bad is happening. "You may not have discomfort as your ears are being damaged," says Patrick Brookhouser, M.D., chairman of the Department of Otolaryngology at Creighton University School of Medicine. "When you get to the point where the noise hurts, you're already way above the damage level."

One sure clue that your environment is too loud is when your hearing temporarily drops a notch. For example, driving home from work, you have to turn up the car radio to hear it; but when you start the car the next morning, you have to fumble quickly to turn down the volume because it seems too loud.

You may also notice these early signs of hearing impairment: ringing or buzzing in your ears, straining to make out muffled speech or an inability to hear a conversation when there's background noise, or difficulty hearing higher-frequency sounds. "When you lose higher frequencies, words sound muffled," says John House, M.D., of the House Ear Institute in Los Angeles. " 'Heat' sounds like 'eat', and 'pin' sounds like 'pen'. And it's not just a matter of turning up the volume with a hearing aid; you're just turning up distorted sound—all bass and no treble."

Thinking about losing your hearing is scary stuff, but noise-related deafness is usually preventable. Here are some ways to take care of your pair:

■ Wear ear protectors while mowing the lawn and operating all power equipment, even a weed trimmer. "Cotton balls or wads of toilet paper won't do," cautions Dr. House. "The plugs should be made of rubber foam or wax, or you should wear acoustic earmuffs." You can buy this ear gear at most pharmacies and gun stores.

■ Earplugs are also a good idea if you're going to a rock concert. (Believe me, you'll still be able to hear the music just fine. But if you want to be a purist about it, get yourself a pair of ER-15

Filtered Earplugs, which soften sounds without blocking any frequencies. According to the manufacturer, the custom-molded earplugs are being worn by a range of performers, from members of the U.S. Air Force Academy Band to the Grateful Dead and Metallica. They cost about $120 a pair. For more information, write: Westone Laboratories, P.O. Box 15100, Colorado Springs, CO 80935.) You'll also want to protect your ears at air shows, car races, tractor pulls, and any other place that's likely to be very noisy.

■ Try not to run more than one appliance at a time. Vacuuming the kitchen floor while your wife operates the food blender subjects you to the noise level of an air-raid siren.

■ Don't smoke or hang out in smoky places. Carbon monoxide, a component of cigarette smoke, restricts the flow of oxygen to nerve cells in the inner ear. A combination of smoking and loud noise is especially hard on hearing. A test of aerospace factory workers found that those who smoked had considerably greater hearing damage than those who didn't.

■ Go easy on the alcohol, too. It can damage the muscles that protect the inner ear from noise.

■ Beware of personal stereos—they can easily put out 100 decibels. Tests have shown that most of the units costing $100 or more are not safe at two-thirds volume.

Wearing headphones while jogging or doing other exercises is even worse, says Los Angeles audiologist Richard Navarro, Ph.D. "Noise triggers a release of adrenaline, which constricts the blood supply to your ears and diverts it to the arms, legs, and heart," he explains. "On top of that, aerobic exercise also diverts blood from the ears to those same muscles. The one-two punch of loud music *and* less blood destroys cilia. It doubles the risk of hearing loss."

■ Get a test to catch any hearing problems early. "Have a hearing test whenever you go to the doctor," says Dr. James Donaldson. "If a hearing loss is detected early, we can save what hearing you have left, at least by convincing you to wear ear protectors."

Dial-a-Hearing-Screening Test offers a free over-the-phone hearing test and referrals to local specialists. For the test number in your area, call (800) 222-3277 or, in Pennsylvania, (800) 345-3277. The self-scored test involves listening to a range of recorded tones. (This service is not available in all areas.)

By being aware of the fragility of your inner ears, and by taking precautions to turn down the volume in your life, you'll retain your good hearing. If you fear you've already blown it, consult an oto-laryngologist (a physician who specializes in hearing problems) to discuss the options, including the possibility of a hearing aid. The newest versions, like the one Ronald Reagan wore throughout his presidency, are so small they're almost impossible to detect, even if you're no longer a rock-and-roll animal and your hair's cut short.

—*David Cardinal*

Part 8

LOOKING GOOD

Hair Care 101

If shinier, cleaner, healthier hair is what you're after, read this chapter. Let the experts teach you a thing or two about good-looking locks.

••••••••••••••••••••••

GUYS AREN'T SUPPOSED to care about their hair. We know this; you know this; shampoo companies know this. To think about such things would be an admission of vanity. Most men would sooner confess that they voted for Richard Nixon (twice) than acknowledge that they give more than an occasional passing thought to their looks.

So admit nothing. Just read on, out of idle curiosity, as we explain how a *theoretical* head of hair might be made to look consistently shiny, clean, and healthy. You don't have to worry about what it means to be learning this stuff, since, if you recall, you never asked.

CLEANLINESS IS NEXT TO NOTHING

We'll start with shine. Shine is directly related to the health and cleanliness of each hair's outer layer, called the cuticle. Seven layers of clear cuticle cells help keep harmful chemicals from penetrating the inner core of the hair and causing damage. The cuticle also holds in moisture needed to keep hair supple. Healthy cuticle cells lie flat, overlapping slightly, like shingles on a roof. When light hits them, it's reflected smoothly, creating shine. Anything that scatters the reflection or dulls the cuticle lessens the gleam.

• •

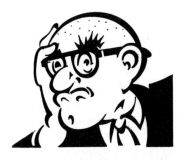

Bald Pills?

Doctors rarely mention baldness as a potential side effect, but a surprising number of popular medications can cause temporary hair loss. Here are just a few:

■ The cholesterol-lowering drugs Atromid-S (clofibrate) and Lopid (gemfibrozil)

■ Many arthritis medications, including Ridaura (auranofin), Indocin (indomethacin), Naprosyn (naproxen), and Clinoril (sulindac)

■ Beta-blocker blood pressure drugs such as tenormin (Atenolol), lopressor (Metroprolol), corgard (Nadolol), and inderal (Propranolol)

■ Anabolic steroids

■ Vitamin-A derived drugs, including Accutane (isotetinoin) and Tegison (etretinate)

Next time your doctor prescribes a drug for you, ask if it's linked to hair loss. Or look it up yourself. An excellent resource is *The Complete Drug Reference,* published by Consumer Reports Books.

The cuticle can be damaged by any number of things—sweat, dust, dirt, heat, solar radiation, chlorine, and air pollution. When this happens, the cells lift like shingles in a storm, and the roughed-up surfaces don't reflect light in the same direction. The result is dull-looking, and often hopelessly tangled, hair.

The solution can be as simple as choosing the right shampoo. The average has 15 ingredients, formulated to clean hair without drying it out. (Some experts believe that the more ingredients a shampoo contains, the better it is.) The cleansing action of a shampoo is provided by a group of cosmetic ingredients called *surfactants,* a fancy name for detergents that loosen oil, dirt, dead cells, and other debris so that they can be rinsed away easily. By combining the right surfactants with other cosmetic ingredients, a basic cleansing shampoo can be developed for oily, normal, or dry hair. (Despite some claims, there's no such thing as a "self-adjusting" shampoo that's right for all types of hair.)

Start by looking for a reputable brand that states on the label that it's for your hair type," says John Corbett, Ph.D., vice president

● ●

Save Your Skin

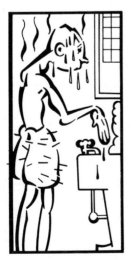

If your skin tends to be dry to begin with, don't aggravate things by taking very hot showers or baths, advises dermatologist Dennis Weigand, M.D., of the University of Oklahoma Health Sciences Center. "The temperature of the water correlates to the drying-out effect," he says. "I tell people who have dry skin to cool their bath water down if it's more than lukewarm." Dr. Weigand says the type of soap you use on dry skin isn't important, but how much you use is: "In general, much more damage is done to the skin from trying to be too clean rather than from not being clean enough."

● ●

DO THICKENING SHAMPOOS WORK?

No shampoo or over-the-counter lotion can slow, halt, or reverse hair loss. However, thickening shampoos and conditioners can make what you have *look* like more. They do this by coating hair shafts with balsam, polymers, or proteins to make hair appear thicker; in some cases, they actually swell individual hairs. Look for terms like *body-building, thickening,* or *volumizing* on the label.

These products are most effective for men whose hair is fine or in the early to middle stages of thinning. Try a few brands until you find one that seems to make a difference for you.

Some hair-styling aids, such as sprays, mousses, and gel dressings, can also make hair look fuller, but beware of using them too often. They can make hair sticky, brittle, and easy to break, which sort of defeats the purpose if you're already losing it.

● ●

of technology at Clairol, Inc. "But there's no single surfactant that's the best for everyone with your hair type. So you may have to try a few before you find which works best for you."

You'll also want to look for a shampoo that's pH-balanced (meaning a pH between 5 and 6). A shampoo with a pH below 5 is too acid and won't lather well, and lathering action is essential for removing dirt and dust.

If you swim in pools regularly, you may need to use a shampoo that's formulated to remove chlorine from the hair. There are several brands available, among them UltraSwim, Revitalize, and Swimmer.

THERE'S OIL IN THEM THERE HAIRS

Excessive oiliness is a common problem, particularly among men with blond hair. "The texture of your hair makes a difference. Oil wicks onto fine, straight hair very easily. But wiry hair doesn't seem oily. It has a lot to do with perception," says Thomas Goodman, Jr., M.D., an assistant professor of dermatology at the University of Tennessee Center for Health Sciences. Men with oily hair should wash it every day, but avoid creamy shampoos that leave behind a heavy residue, which can weigh down oily hair. A post-shampoo rinse with a solution of 1 teaspoon of vinegar in a pint of water can also help remove soap residues.

To the age-old question of whether to lather up and rinse once or twice when shampooing, there's no universal answer. In most cases, one round will do the trick; but if you have oily hair, work outdoors, or live in a big city, you may have to suds up again to get your hair completely clean. Oily hair may need more cleaning in the summer, when heat and humidity step up the production of sweat and oil on the scalp.

Shampooing is only the first step. To get hair really shiny, you need a conditioner. Conditioners contain ingredients that fill in nicks on the hair shaft and smooth the cuticle. They also cut down the amount of static in your hair. Static keeps hairs from lying smoothly together and allows them to tangle more readily, reducing shine. "Your hair naturally has a lot of negative ionic charges along the shaft," says Rebecca Caserio, M.D., clinical assistant professor of dermatology at the University of Pittsburgh. "This causes static. Conditioners add a positive charge, which helps neutralize the static."

"When the hairs lie together better," explains Dr. John Corbett, "shine from one hair is reinforced by that of the adjacent hair. What the eye perceives as shine is actually groups of hairs lying parallel to one another to reflect the light."

Conditioners not only help protect hair from outside assaults; they also repair existing damage. But there are genuine differences among the ingredients used in conditioners. "If your hair is already damaged, it's especially important to choose a conditioner that will counteract the specific problem," says Dr. Corbett. For example, if your hair is very dry, try conditioners with small amounts of oil in them. (Look on the label for dimethicone or mineral oil.) For fine hair, select a conditioner with a watery consistency, such as a spray-on type that you leave on the hair.

There are two main ways to go about conditioning your hair: using a combination "conditioning shampoo," and using a separate conditioner. Conditioning shampoos, which combine the two functions in one product, work best for people whose hair isn't heavily damaged. (If you swim in pools a lot, work outdoors, or live in a large city, that probably excludes you.) The advantage of conditioning shampoos is that they're convenient. The disadvantage is that they neither clean as well as plain cleansing shampoos nor condition as well as separate conditioners.

A good compromise is to alternate. Try using a basic cleansing shampoo for every third or fourth washing and a conditioning shampoo the rest of the time.

DRY FACTS ABOUT DRY HAIR

If your hair is damaged, dry, or prone to tangles, you probably need to use a separate conditioner all the time. Just remember that conditioners are formulated to cling to the hair shaft and not be rinsed away. With repeated use, this film can build up and attract dirt, leaving your hair looking limp. The problem is even worse if you use hair sprays and other styling aids, says Dr. Rebecca Caserio. However, occasional use of a plain shampoo—and no conditioner—can keep this buildup from becoming a problem.

Another thing to look for is heat damage, so go easy with that blow dryer. Overdrying evaporates the water in the hair shaft that keeps it strong and pliable. To blow-dry for minimum damage and maximum shine:

- Towel-dry hair before you blow-dry. It's faster and easier on your hair.
- Use your blow dryer on a low heat setting.
- Hold it at least 6 inches from your head.
- Keep the dryer moving so the air flow isn't directed at the same spot for more than a few seconds.
- Gently finger-comb your hair while it's drying to prevent tangles.
- The top layer of your hair is particularly susceptible to overdrying because it takes the most abuse from the weather. Stop before this area is bone-dry.

That's all you need to know to keep your hair looking clean and shiny all the time . . . or should we say, to keep your *theoretical* hair clean and shiny all the time.

—William Harnham

Fill 'Er Up

Smile. When it comes to fixing cavities,
picking the right fillin' isn't so chillin'.
Here's some helpful information to chew on.

• • • • • • • • • • • • • • • • • • • •

IF YOU'RE LIKE MOST guys, you don't have the slightest idea
what kind of fillings your dentist puts in your mouth. He probably
assumes you want the same type that's already in there, not realizing that when you had those teeth filled at 18, you were more interested in sneaking a peek at his assistant's cleavage than you were in
what was going into that cavity in your third molar.

Well, you're a big boy now, and it's time you sat up in the dentist's chair and paid a little more attention. There's more than one
way to fill a tooth. In fact, nowadays you have at least four choices:
silver, gold, composite, and porcelain. The following guide—plus a
healthy dose of advice from your dentist—can help you decide
which is right for you.

SILVER

Silver is the workhorse of the bunch—it's been used far more
often than any other filling material. And that's not surprising, since
it was introduced more than 150 years ago. With that kind of history,
it's no wonder dentists have a lot of faith in it. It's effective, easy for
dentists to apply, and lasts for decades. It's also the least expensive
of all the options.

Silver offers durability for high-stress areas like the back of the
mouth, where biting force is greatest. It does tend to darken,
though, so it may not be the best choice cosmetically for the front of
the mouth.

These fillings are actually made from a combination of metals,
including silver, copper, tin, and mercury. The more proper name
for this material is amalgam, but it's commonly called silver because
of its color.

There is some controversy over the possibility that mercury
might leak out of these fillings and harm people. (Mercury is toxic
when ingested in high amounts.) At least one study has shown that

mercury from silver fillings can cause kidney malfunction in test animals. The American Dental Association (ADA), however, says there's "no reason for the public to be concerned."

A handful of dentists have tried to capitalize on the mercury scare by offering to replace silver fillings. Unless your fillings are cracked or discolored and need replacement, there's no reason to subject yourself to this. In fact, removing a mouthful of perfectly good fillings holds the potential for tooth damage.

GOLD

Fillings made from this precious metal are also very durable, making it another good choice for the back of the mouth. Gold is especially useful for restoring teeth that have very large cavities. Such teeth are prone to cracking, and since gold fillings don't expand and contract with temperature changes as silver fillings do, they're less likely to cause a tooth to crack. In fact, gold is sometimes used to surround the outside of a tooth to prevent it from breaking. A softer filling, gold will not wear down the opposing teeth (as porcelain can). Finally, gold fillings last even longer than silver.

With this extra dependability, however, comes a bigger price tag. Depending on the size and location of the filling, gold can cost three to six times as much as silver. All of the extra cost may not be covered by your insurance, so you might want to check before you go for the gold.

COMPOSITE

These quartz/acrylic fillings are an appealing option for the front of your mouth because they can be colored to match your tooth enamel and blend in with your smile.

They haven't been around as long as gold and silver, though, so dentists aren't yet sure how long they last. The older composite fillings did have a tendency toward long-term "microleakage" (so small you can't see it), which could lead to decay under the filling. But the newer-generation composites bond more closely to the tooth and have much less of a leakage problem.

Composites are more susceptible to being worn down by opposing teeth, making them less desirable for back teeth. And solvents like alcohol and vinegar may weaken the composite.

For front teeth, the less durable but cosmetically agreeable composite may be a good choice. Composites are slightly more expensive than silver fillings.

PORCELAIN

Often lumped into a "white filling" category with composites, porcelain is actually a more durable cosmetic filling. Unlike composites, porcelain fillings do not wear down easily. But they are more abrasive toward opposing teeth than any other filling, "so your dentist may advise against them in areas where they would directly wear on other teeth or softer fillings," says Barry Dale, D.M.D., a spokesman for the Academy of General Dentistry.

Porcelain fillings are also more expensive than composites. Their higher price comes from the two-day procedure it takes to place them in the tooth. They're used most often in back teeth, especially those that show when you smile.

—Greg Gutfeld

Smooth Strokes

*Avoiding razor nicks is a matter of sharp skills.
Tape these tips on your bathroom mirror.*

●●●●●●●●●●●●●●●●●●●●●

AL'S BEARD IS COSTING me money. At the poker table last week, I was thinking to myself that nothing's more irritating than trying to read his (formerly) expressive face now that he has this thick growth of ugly whiskers covering everything. I was looking at his up cards, wondering whether he'd pulled the case ace. Used to be, a little crease would form off to the side of his lip that would betray him. No more. I've had to resort to playing the cards.

In fairness to Al, however, maybe one thing's more irritating: the thing that brought on the beard in the first place. Turns out, a dermatologist told him he needed a beard to cure a bad case of ingrown hairs.

Technically, his condition is called *pseudofolliculitis barbae,* but "razor bumps" will do. It's the most common of many causes of inflamed hair follicles in men—especially black men. The painful bumps develop when the razor-sharpened tips of curly whiskers arc back to the skin and grow inward. "Once the hair comes back into the skin, it's attacked by the body's natural defenses just as any foreign body is, setting the stage for painful infections," says skin-care maven Lia Schorr, author of *Lia Schorr's Skin Care Guide for Men.*

One way to ward off the dreaded bumps is to do like Al and grow a beard, but that's rather extreme. Often a slight modification in your shaving regimen will do the trick. Men are encouraged to think a good shave means making the skin as smooth as a baby's behind, but the best thing for your skin may actually be *not* to shave that closely. "The closer you shave, the more you may encourage ingrown hairs, as only very short hairs can reenter the skin once they've come out," says Schorr.

These shaving tips may help prevent damage and keep things more comfortable.

DON'T . . .

- Shave against the grain of your beard. This encourages hairs to be clipped below the skin's surface, where they can curve back and pierce the wall of the hair follicle.
- Stretch your skin taut while going over it with the blade. "When the skin is released, the short hairs pull back below the surface," says Jerome Litt, M.D., author of *Your Skin: From Acne to Zits.*
- Shave over an area more than twice. "No one will be examining your skin with a magnifying glass," says Lia Schorr.
- Shave right before you exercise: Sweat irritates newly shaven skin.

DO . . .

- Go gently. A good shave doesn't have to do violence to your skin.
- Shave after showering, so your face is as moist as possible. Otherwise, soak your beard for 2 minutes in hot, soapy water.
- Soften your face for 2 more minutes with shaving cream.
- Replace your blade often.

■ Start at the upper cheeks and move down, thus exposing the beard's toughest areas to the cream's softening benefits longest.

Still, that's all preventive medicine. What if you've already got those nasty little bumps? Dr. Litt says you have to stop shaving for a few days at least. This gives the hairs that have looped back into your skin a chance to grow out—and it gives your skin a rest from the daily grind. Yes, the Don Johnson look went out a few years ago, but your skin doesn't care about fashion.

There is another alternative, but it's only for those who are truly dedicated. You can lift out those little ingrown-hair loops with a beard pick—a device with a sharp, curved tip—available at barber-supply stores. Try the Moore Technique Shaving System, designed by dermatologist Milton Moore, M.D. It comes with a preshave lubricant, anti-inflammatory cream, antibacterial cream, and a beard pick. You'll find it at many drugstores and some beauty salons—$15.95 for a two-month supply. Order from Moore Innovations, Inc., P.O. Box 300445, Houston, TX 77230.

Dr. Litt also advises using a warm, wet washcloth to bring the bumps to a head, then plucking out the hairs with sterile tweezers. If you do this, yank in the direction of the growth. If you can't get it in two tries, give up: Digging around with the tweezers can irritate or inflame the skin. Al tried this approach and indeed found it made his skin more irritated. He was desperate, so he just grew the damn beard.

Fortunately, this wasn't a problem at his job; but it is for some men who grow beards and even for many who shave just every other day, says Robert Fitzpatrick, a Washington, D.C., attorney who cofounded the PFB (*Pseudofolliculitis barbae*) Project "to fight job discrimination against bearded men." Fitzpatrick considers PFB a "societal disease" because pressure forces men with curly hair to shave clean. (For more information, write PFB Project, 4801 Massachusetts Avenue NW, Suite 400, Washington, DC 20016-2087.)

Of course, rules about shaving aren't a problem if folliculitis crops up elsewhere on the body. Although razor bumps are the most common form of folliculitis, the pinhead-sized yellow pustules can occur almost anywhere on the skin, says Richard Refowich, M.D., head of dermatology at St. Luke's Hospital in Bethlehem, Pennsylvania. For instance, they can result from bacteria picked up while soaking in hot tubs. Washing afterward with an antibacterial soap helps prevent infections. Topical antibiotics containing bacitracin or neomycin will usually clear them up, Dr. Refowich says.

I have another friend, Howie, who complains about ingrown hairs. I explained all the options. When I finally came to the easiest solution, he said, "No way." He's proud of his face, he told me. That was a month ago. Now his beard is making him uglier by the day.

—Richard Laliberte

Hide Your Hide

Who says there's no effortless way to slim down? Choosing the right wardrobe can make you look 10 pounds lighter.

• • • • • • • • • • • • • • • • • • • •

Forget about throwing your weight around at the office. In the business world, a pudgy profile makes you appear sloppy and disorganized—as though you lack self-control. In fact, studies show that thinner executives typically earn about $3,000 a year more than their heavier counterparts for doing the same work.

If you can't lose those stubborn extra few pounds, you still can avoid receiving a thinner paycheck by *looking* trimmer in the way you dress. Here's how.

Create vertical lines. Pinstripes are perfect. They draw the eye in a natural up-and-down direction, emphasizing height over width. Similarly, subtle or small patterns make you look taller than bold or big patterns, which break up the line of the body and seem to add bulk.

Dressing vertically also means wearing shirts and trousers that don't contrast. The eye stops at the boundary between a stark white shirt and black pants. Instead wear a gray shirt, so the vertical flow is uninterrupted.

Forget bow ties—that wide expanse of shirt underneath them just showcases your spare tire. Wear long ties, the tip of which should touch the top to middle of your belt. (A short tie resting on your stomach may prompt unwanted comparisons between you and Lou Costello.)

Wear cool colors. Black, charcoal gray, and navy, aside from being classic suit colors that command authority, actually distance you from your observers and tend to unload some cargo. "Dark, cool, muted colors in a suit can make you appear 10 to 15 pounds slimmer," says image consultant Lois Fenton, author of *Dress for Excellence*. In sportswear, blue and green will also have slimming power. Conversely, steer clear of warm hues like red, yellow, and orange. These colors bring you closer and bulk you up.

Beware of flashy clothes. For you, the sharkskin suit is a killing machine. Loud, shiny, or bright colors draw all eyes to you and accentuate your width. If you love bright colors, save them for accents. It's fine to wear a tie and braces in startling hues. Under a gray or navy suit, a red or yellow tie will actually draw favorable attention to your face, fashion consultants say.

● ●

Pardon Your Parents

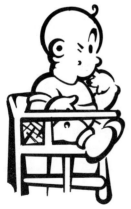

Genes make a convenient scapegoat for a host of inadequacies. Unfortunately, fat is no longer one of them. According to Duke University researchers who analyzed data from several studies, only thinness is inherited. When Danish and American scientists compared adopted children with their biological and adoptive parents, the obese kids were no more likely to have fat biological parents than they were to have fat adoptive parents. Only when the researchers looked at skinny offspring did they find a connection. Thin children were significantly less likely to have overweight parents—whether they were compared with their mother, father, or both.

Wear light- to medium-weight fabrics. Heavyweight garments exaggerate girth. The best materials for slimming effect: twills, gabardines, and thin-wale corduroys. Leave bulky Harris tweeds to underfed professors.

Stay loose. Avoid close-fitting clothes; they emphasize bulges. It's particularly important that the upper chest, shoulders, and upper sleeves of your jackets not be tight. Tight fabric there will stretch, wrinkle, and bulge, producing a corrugated look.

Some final tips:

■ If you're wide in the derriere, avoid ventless jackets. These tend to ride up in back, creating an effect about equal to wearing a sign that says "Kick me." If your weight is in your torso, a ventless jacket can have a slimming effect, although some heavy men find ventless jackets less comfortable than those with center or side vents.

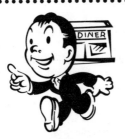

Walk Home from the Restaurant

Should you heed Mom's warning and wait for an hour after lunch before diving in with your new fins? Not necessarily. Mild exercise can actually aid the digestive process. But there's another good reason to time your workouts carefully around meals: weight loss.

According to Bryant Stamford, Ph.D., director of the Health Promotion and Wellness Center and professor of allied health in the School of Medicine at the University of Louisville, mild exercise after eating can engage something called the *thermic effect*. Dr. Stamford reported in *Physician and Sportsmedicine* that the energy required to digest food can be *doubled* with mild exercise after a meal.

But a major workout is better taken before a meal—for a couple of reasons. First, your metabolic rate stays up for some time after exercise, resulting in an afterburn that uses calories. Perhaps more important, vigorous exercise reduces your body's glycogen (sugar) stores. So carbohydrates you eat will simply replace the ones you burned off instead of being turned to fat. The final word: Exercise may also reduce your appetite.

■ Be careful with pleats. If they fit just right, pleated pants can hide a multitude of sins, but if you wear them too tight or if you're very large in the belly, the pleats will stand out, making you look like a fan. Generally, the wider the pleat, the less likely it is to spread apart.

■ Cuffs shorten legs and accentuate body width.

■ For the beefy, barrel-chested man, the double row of buttons on double-breasted jackets cuts away thickness.

■ Select shirts with button-down or standard collars rather than "wide load" spread collars.

—*Jennifer Whitlock*

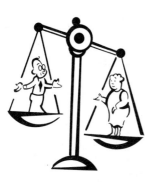

The Male Advantage

Male smokers who quit don't gain as much weight as women, reports *The New England Journal of Medicine.* A decade-long study of 9,000 adults finds that men only gain about 6 pounds on average– 2 pounds less than women gain. Another surprising finding: The average smoker weighs less than a nonsmoker, so quitting only brings you back to your normal weight.

Part 9

BOD LIKE A ROCK

Make Gains Fast

Get the ultimate workout in just 40 minutes.
Dozens of top exercise experts tell you how to squeeze
the most pump into the least amount of time.

●●●●●●●●●●●●●●●●●●●●●

IF YOU WANT STRONGER muscles, a better body, and more speed and endurance but aren't doing anything to get them, we bet we know why: no time. There's the job, the business trips, the family, the friends, the yard chores, the civic club, the newspapers and trade journals. You have the best of intentions, but you also have a very full dance card.

Well, we're here to say you can make your fitness goals and have a life, too. All you have to do is find a measly 40 minutes, three times a week. That's long enough to get your heart and muscles pumping and short enough to stave off boredom, and it fits neatly into a lunch hour with some time to spare.

The secret of fast fitness is efficiency. *Men's Health* consulted dozens of top exercise physiologists, coaches, and professional athletes to help us create short, targeted workouts for every man—whether your goal is muscle growth, weight loss, or general fitness.

Consistency is the key to success. You'll get the fastest results if you follow a Monday-Wednesday-Friday routine. "A man begins to lose the strength and endurance benefits he's gained from his exercise program after 60 hours away from the gym," says Charles Kuntzleman, Ed.D., national program director for Fitness Finders. "But even a two-day-a-week program is better than no program at all."

Each of these workout programs should begin with a warm-up and end with a cool-down. The warm-up—essentially some calisthenics or light aerobic activity like brisk walking or stationary cycling, followed by some stretching—allows your muscles, heart, and lungs to ease into the session without shocking your system. The cool-down takes your body back to a resting state more gradually. When you stop short, your heart rate and blood pressure plummet, which can cause feelings of light-headedness or dizziness. Winding down slowly also helps to clear lactic acid, a by-product of intense exercise, out of your bloodstream. Some experts believe that lactic acid is responsible for delayed-onset muscle soreness—that achy feeling that strikes the day after a workout. Stretching is also important; it keeps muscles limber and reduces the risk of injury.

For guidance on the correct form for the exercises that follow, check with the fitness instructor at your health club, try a session with a personal trainer, or check out one of these books: *Getting Stronger,* by Bill Pearl and Gary T. Moran; *The Complete Book of Nautilus Training,* by Michael D. Wolf; and *Home Gym Fitness: Free Weight Workouts,* by Charles T. Kuntzleman.

Before starting, you'll need to know a few numbers. First figure out your maximum heart rate (max H.R.): max H.R. = 220 − your age. Next determine your correct heart-rate training range. This depends on your exercise goals.

For example, A 40-year-old man on the Fat Burner program would first calculate his maximum heart rate (220 − 40 = 180); then he would look up the desired training range for that workout. In his case, it's 60 to 70 percent of his maximum heart rate. So to get the desired benefits, he should try to keep his heart rate between 108 (0.60 × 180) and 126 (0.70 × 180) beats per minute.

To calculate your pulse rate, press lightly with two fingers on your wrist or neck, count the number of beats you feel in 10 seconds, and multiply that number by 6. For constant feedback on your intensity level, try a heart-rate monitor. The new models are an amazingly accurate and reasonably priced way to keep tabs on your workouts—some models even offer computer hookups that allow you to graph your fitness progress.

Here are our programs. (Do check with your doctor before proceeding.)

GENERAL FITNESS ROUTINE

This plan is perfect for the man who's just starting to exercise or who doesn't have any specific exercise goals other than to look and feel better. It provides a solid strength and endurance base. If you're out of shape, you should start here, even though compet-

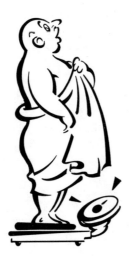

Slow Down, Big Guy

Exercise is a good way to lose weight, but many men get stuck about 5 pounds shy of their target. Logic tells us to exercise harder to break this plateau, but a Yale psychologist specializing in obesity suggests a better tactic: He explains that losing too much weight too fast may force the body into a "defensive mode," lowering its metabolic rate. To shed the last few pounds, "try decreasing activity to a reasonable level to give the body a chance to adjust," says Kelly Brownell, Ph.D.

ing in the Ironman may be your ultimate goal. After about eight weeks on this program, you'll be ready to start one of the more advanced ones.

Monday and Friday

Start: Warm-up #1 (see "Warm-Ups" on page 208), 5 minutes.

Middle: Fifteen minutes of continuous aerobic exercise (60 to 70 percent of max H.R.) such as brisk walking, running, biking, stair climbing, cross-country skiing, or rowing, followed by 15 minutes of weight training using either machines or free weights.

Do the exercises below in order, in a circuit fashion—performing one complete set of eight to ten repetitions and then moving to the next. Rest 30 seconds between stations. In 15 minutes, you should be able to do two complete circuits. For each machine, start with a weight that allows you to do ten easy repetitions. Once you're comfortable with your form, increase the weight (one notch or plate on exercise machines, 5 pounds with free weights) every other workout until you reach the maximum weight you can lift for that exercise and still complete ten repetitions for each of two sets.

Exercise Stations: Leg extension, leg curl, low back machine, bench press, lat pulldown, military press, tricep pushdown, bicep curl.

Finish: Cool-down #1 (see "Cool-Downs" on page 209), 5 minutes.

Wednesday

Start: Warm-up #1 (see "Warm-Ups" on page 208), 5 minutes.

Middle: A 30-minute aerobic circuit. This should be done just like the circuit program on Monday and Friday, with a single significant exception: *Replace the 30 seconds of rest between sets with 30 seconds of aerobic exercise.* For example, when you get off the bench press machine, immediately hop on a stationary cycle, jump rope, or run in place before moving on to flies. Eliminating the rest period and adding aerobic activity between sets allows you to get an aerobic workout while weight lifting. Do two circuits, each consisting of the following exercises.

Exercise Stations: Leg extension, leg press, leg curl, calf raise, low back machine or hyperextensions, push-up, bench press, fly, military press, lateral raise, upright row, pull-up, lat pulldown, tricep pushdown, bicep curl.

Finish: Cool-down #1 (see "Cool-Downs" on page 209), 5 minutes.

●●

WARM-UPS

To help ready your muscles for more strenuous activity, do these warm-ups as indicated in the exercise routines described in this chapter.

#1

Use this warm-up for all aerobic-related routines:

■ Three minutes of gentle aerobic exercise, doing a scaled-down version of the activity you'll perform in the main part of the routine. For example, if you're going to run, walk briskly or jog; if you're going to use the stair climber, set the machine about half as high as you will during the main part of the exercise.

■ Two minutes of stretching, concentrating on the muscles you're going to use or on those that feel especially tight. For example, if you're going to ride a bike, pay particular attention to your quads and your lower back; if you plan to run, key on hamstrings and calves.

#2

■ Three minutes of gentle aerobic exercise, doing a scaled-down version of the same activity you'll perform in the main part of the routine.

■ Two minutes of stretching, concentrating on the muscles you're going to use in the main part of the workout.

■ Five minutes of moderate aerobic activity such as brisk walking, running, biking, stair climbing, cross-country skiing, or rowing.

#3

■ Three minutes of calisthenics, consisting of two sets of push-ups and two sets of sit-ups or crunches.

■ Two minutes of stretching, concentrating on the muscles you're going to use or on those that feel especially tight. Note: Stretching can be done between sets to loosen up particular muscles before or after they have been worked.

●●

THE FAT BURNER

Got a couple of stubborn pounds sitting around your midsection that you'd like to lose? This is the program for you. Burning fat is actually easier than most people think. It doesn't require long, painful hours in the gym or the humiliation of being wrapped in

● ●

COOL-DOWNS

Cool-down is an important component of any workout; be sure to do these routines as advised in this chapter.

#1

■ Two sets of sit-ups or crunches.
■ Three minutes of stretching, concentrating on muscles worked in the session or on those that feel especially tight.

#2

■ Two minutes of gentle aerobic exercise, doing a scaled-down version of the same activity performed in the main part of the routine.
■ One set of sit-ups or crunches.
■ One set on the low back machine.
■ Two minutes of stretching, concentrating on muscles worked in the session or on those that feel especially tight.

#3

■ Five minutes of moderate aerobic activity—whatever you were doing in the main part of the routine.
■ Five minutes of stretching.

● ●

plastic and trundled off to a steam room. "Consistency and moderate aerobic exercise are the keys to losing weight," says Stu Mittleman, a personal trainer and owner of New York Ultrafit, a center for fitness evaluations and personal training. "Choose exercises that you enjoy and can sustain for 20 to 30 minutes of continuous activity three times a week."

Monday and Friday

Start: Warm-up #1 (see "Warm-Ups" on the opposite page), 5 minutes.

Middle: Thirty minutes of continuous aerobic exercise (60 to 70 percent of max H.R.) such as brisk walking, running, biking, stair climbing, cross-country skiing, or rowing.

Finish: Cool-down #2 (see "Cool-Downs" above), 5 minutes.

Wednesday

Start: Warm-up #1 (see "Warm-Ups" on the opposite page), 5 minutes.

Middle: Thirty minutes of aerobic exercise (60 to 75 percent of max H.R.). Switch exercises every 5 to 10 minutes. For example, do 5 minutes on the stationary bike, 5 minutes on the rowing machine, 5 minutes on the treadmill, 5 minutes on the stair climber, 5 minutes on the cross-country ski machine, 5 minutes jumping rope. (If you don't have a wide variety of equipment available, alternate between bench stepping, rope jumping, and jogging in place.)

Finish: Cool-down #2 (see "Cool-Downs" on page 209), 5 minutes.

ENDURANCE BUILDER

To increase endurance, you'll have to turn up the volume. "Moderately-paced exercise is fine for burning calories, but when you want to build your endurance, you have to work at a slightly higher intensity level," says Budd Coates, exercise physiologist and world-class marathoner. "Over time, your cardiovascular system adapts to the added stress, making you more efficient and letting you go longer and farther with less effort."

Monday, Wednesday, and Friday

Start: Warm-up #1 (see "Warm-Ups" on page 208), 5 minutes.

Middle: Thirty minutes of continuous aerobic exercise (70 to 80 percent of max H.R.). Use any exercises you like, such as brisk walking, running, biking, stair climbing, cross-country skiing, or rowing, so long as you maintain your target heart rate.

• •

The Early Edge

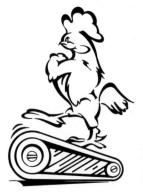

Exercise early, and you exercise better. A study pitting morning exercisers against evening exercisers found that early birds came to classes more frequently and were less likely to drop out than the late crowd. It's largely a practical matter, according to the study's authors. At the start of the day, you're less likely to have a schedule conflict. Those who find themselves frequently putting off their workouts might benefit from a switch to the uncluttered morning time slot.

You may use different machines on different days, but remain on one machine during a single exercise session. It's very difficult to maintain an intensity level of 70 to 80 percent of max H.R. while changing machines.

If you can't stay at this level for the full 30 minutes (and you won't be able to at first), it's okay to reduce the intensity until you get your breath back (about 3 minutes). Then if you feel better, up the intensity to your target zone. Use as many recovery slowdowns as you need to get through the 30 minutes, but keep going and keep trying to get your heart rate back up into the training range. As your body adapts, your endurance will improve, and you will need fewer breaks.

Finish: Cool-down #2 (see "Cool-Downs" on page 209), 5 minutes.

SPEED BUILDER

In a hurry? Whether you're preparing for a race or just looking to get a step ahead of the competition in your racquetball game, this workout's for you. Its high intensity not only gets results but gets them fast. In fact, this is the one workout where we're going to tell you to cut your session short. Go for the burn. Then get back to your office. You can be done in much less time than 40 minutes.

"When you're talking speed or increased performance, you need intervals," says Pat Croce, physical conditioning coach for the Philadelphia Flyers and 76ers. Intervals are repeated short periods of intense exercise (like wind sprints) broken up by light exercise (like jogging in place or bench stepping) for recovery.

Monday and Friday

Follow Monday and Friday "Endurance Builder" program schedule exactly as described. (See the opposite page.)

Wednesday

Start: Warm-up #2 (see "Warm-Ups" on page 208), 10 minutes.

Middle: Five sets consisting of 1 minute of hard aerobic activity (80 to 90 percent of max H.R.) followed by 1 minute of very easy aerobic activity to recover. Some suggested activities: running, race walking, biking, stair climbing, cross-country skiing, or rowing.

Finish: Cool-down #3 (see "Cool-Downs" on page 209), 10 minutes.

MUSCLE TONER

Not all bodybuilders want to look like the Wild Samoan. This program is for a man who seeks more strength and vitality but an overall appearance that's lean and firm, not brawny. Building muscle tone is a careful process of shaping—some might even say sculpting—the muscles. The result is a subtle increase in what bodybuilders call "definition"—the ripple effect. It's a two-pronged effort: part fat burning, part muscle building.

Monday and Friday

Start: Warm-up #3 (see "Warm-Ups" on page 208), 5 minutes.

Middle: Thirty minutes of weight training, using free weights whenever possible. "When building muscle tone, it is important to use lighter weights and do fast-paced repetitions with little rest between sets," says Anthony D. Mahon, Ph.D., of Ball State's Human Performance Laboratory. Use a circuit approach, going from one exercise to the next fairly quickly. The rapid pace adds fat-burning aerobic benefits.

Do the exercises below in order. With each, crank out 10 to 12 repetitions, rest 30 seconds, and then move to the next station. In 30 minutes, you should be able to do two complete circuits. Start with a weight that allows you to do 12 easy repetitions. Once you're comfortable with your form, increase the weight 5 to 10 pounds every other workout until you can do 12 repetitions of the exercise on the first circuit but only 10 on the second. Once your muscles adapt to this new weight and you can blast out 12 repetitions on both circuits, bump the weight up another notch.

Exercise Stations: Leg extension, leg press, leg curl, calf raise, low back machine, bench press with barbell or dumbbells, dumbbell fly, lat pulldown behind the head, military press with barbell or dumbbells, seated row with cables or machine, lateral raise with dumbbells, upright row with barbell or dumbbells, tricep pushdown on machine, bicep curl with barbell or dumbbells, wrist curl with barbell or dumbbells.

Finish: Cool-down #1 (see "Cool-Downs" on page 209), 5 minutes.

Wednesday

Start: Warm-up #3 (see "Warm-Ups" on page 208), 5 minutes.

Middle: A 30-minute circuit program as on Monday and Friday, but with a few modifications. This workout contains fewer exercises, giving you time to do three circuits instead of two. Also, while the Monday and Friday workouts concentrate on free weights, this workout uses machines. Changing to machines will work your muscles at slightly different angles, producing a wider range of strength and better definition. Perform three circuits of 10 to 12 repetitions of each of the following exercises, allowing yourself 30 seconds of rest between sets.

Exercise Stations: Leg extension, leg curl, low back machine, bench press on machine, fly on machine, lat pulldown to chest, military press on machine, lateral raise on machine, tricep kickback, bicep curl on machine.

Finish: Cool-down #1 (see "Cool-Downs" on page 209), 5 minutes.

BODY BLASTER

Size has its benefits. Let's face it: Larger men seem to have a more dominating presence in the world. If you want to make sure nobody ever kicks sand in your face at the beach, this is your program.

Here, the rhythm is quite different from all the other workouts. The pace slows down, and the focus is on volume (pounds lifted), not intensity (speed of the repetitions). "When building muscle, you want to concentrate on overloading the muscle, so you have to use heavier weights than you would if you were going for tone," says Frank Zane, three-time Mr. Universe and three-time Mr. Olympia turned personal trainer.

Further, when size is your goal, it is best to work one body part at a time instead of following a circuit program, so you can really overload the muscle and encourage the most growth. Do all three sets of one exercise before moving on to the next. Take your time. The slow pace will also allow you more rest between sets—and you'll need it so your body can recover for another intense effort.

Monday and Friday

Start: Warm-up #3 (see "Warm-Ups" on page 208), 5 minutes.

Middle: A 30-minute stacked-set weight-training program as described above. Do three sets of each exercise, resting 45 seconds to 1 minute between sets. Increase the weight and decrease the repetitions with each set. On the first set, do 8 to 12 repetitions; on the second, do 6 to 8; on the third, you should be able to complete only 3 to 6.

Exercise Stations: Leg extension, leg press, bench press with barbell or dumbbells, lat pulldown behind the head, military press with barbell, upright row with barbell, tricep pushdown on machine, bicep curl with barbell.

Finish: Cool-down #1 (see "Cool-Downs" on page 209), 5 minutes.

Wednesday

Start: Warm-up #3 (see "Warm-Ups" on page 208), 5 minutes.

Middle: Thirty minutes of weight training, following the same format as on Monday and Friday. Some of the exercises have been replaced with others that work the same muscle group but from a different point of attack. For example, flies have been substituted for bench presses—different exercises, but both targeting the chest muscles. In other exercises, we've simply switched from barbells to dumbbells, once again in an effort to stress the muscle from a slightly different angle.

Exercise Stations: Leg press, leg curl, dumbbell fly, lat pulldown to chest, military press with dumbbells, upright row with dumbbells, tricep kickback, bicep curl with dumbbells.

Finish: Cool-down #1 (see "Cool-Downs" on page 209), 5 minutes.

Now that you know the basic programs, all you have to do is fine-tune them according to your schedule and the equipment available to you. Remember to add variety to your workouts. Trying new exercises or new combinations of exercises will keep you from going stale, both physically and mentally.

Once you've done this, you're left with two choices: Either start building a bigger, faster, healthier body, or use those 40 minutes to come up with another excuse not to exercise.

—Dan Bensimhon

Home Sweat Home

*Why join a health club? A great home gym
can be yours for less than you may think.
Start your shopping here.*

● ●

EVERYONE KNOWS THE advantages of a home workout over a
health-club routine. No drive time. No waiting in line for your (and
everyone else's) favorite machine. No having to deal with conde-
scending looks from loutish guys who can bench-press five times
your weight. And no more sweaty locker rooms.

So why not set up a complete home gym of your own? Time
was, you needed the personal income and the spacious quarters of a
precrash commodities broker to do this properly. That, or settle for
cheaply made equipment that was uncomfortable to use and built to
collapse on set number 27, rep 12. But today, there are lots of manu-
facturers making health club–quality machines for home use that
won't break your budget.

A well-rounded fitness routine has three aspects—cardiovascular conditioning, strength training, and stretching. Of course, you
could accomplish these for no money at all simply by running in
place, doing calisthenics, and then stretching on your living-room
carpet. But having your own gym is something else again. It really is
a powerful incentive to stick with the program.

Men's Health offers the following guide to assembling a complete home gym for under $1,000. After that, we show you what you
can get if your budget is a little bit larger.

THE $1,000 VERSION

Strength equipment—$550 to $650. In this price range,
you'll use free weights—sets of dumbbells, barbells, and a weight
bench—for your strength-training regimen. Many experts believe
pumping free weights is one of the best and fastest ways to build
strength and sculpt the body. Start with a sturdy multipurpose
bench with an adjustable incline, a leg extension/leg curl feature, a
padded arm curl attachment, and a rack for your barbell.

Some benches are designed for add-ons like a dip station, a lat pulldown, or butterfly. These accessories are nice extras for rounding out your routine. For an all-in-one weight bench, check out the BodySmith Workout Center by ParaBody (about $350). Excel and Marcy Fitness Products also offer good values in benches in about the same price range, depending on accessories.

As for weights, a 110-pound set is a good starting place. Serious lifters usually prefer Olympic-style weights (with the large holes in the center and larger barbell), but standard weights work just as well. Figure on paying $1 per pound. You can also find some 310-pound Olympic weight sets for under $200.

Cardiovascular equipment—$300 to $450. You'll find several models of stationary bikes, stair climbers, and cross-country ski machines in this price range. Your first choice is deciding which machine suits you best.

If you are buying a stationary bike, be certain it has a secure-locking, comfortable seat, adjustable handlebars, smooth pedaling action, and digital performance feedback for time, speed, and distance. Look for the bike that has the most solid construction and feels the best when you're on it. The Tunturi Executive Ergometer ($299) and Bodyguard's 955 (about $350) are both good bets.

Stair climbers have become very popular in the last two years because they provide not only good aerobic exercise but also excellent lower-body conditioning. Again, solid construction and frame stability are the key factors. You should also demand smooth stepping action. In the $350 to $450 range, you'll find several models

· ·

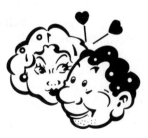

Hubbies on the Run

You're more likely to keep to an exercise routine if you work out with your wife, according to a study of attendance at a thrice-weekly fitness program. Only 10 percent of married couples dropped out before the end of the program. The dropout rate was 22 percent for men who attended without their wives.

that are solidly built and offer feedback on time, step rate, and total steps taken. Precor's 718e, which was one of the first stair climbers designed for home use, is still about the best value for around $400. You can save about $50 by opting for the 714, which is the same basic unit as the 718e but without the electronic feedback.

Cross-country ski machines simultaneously work the lower and upper body while improving cardiovascular conditioning. Unfortunately, the $59 wonder machines advertised on TV just don't hold up with regular use. Look for units with solid construction, smooth sliding action for legs, and independent movement of the arm levers. A great new unit for about $300 is the FM320 by Fitness Master: It's smooth, easy to use, and aesthetically appealing. NordicTrack is the original maker of cross-country ski machines, and its line of products is extensive. The NordicTrack 303 ($399) is solidly built and a fine value as well.

Stretching—total cost, $50 to $150. You don't need any equipment for stretching, but you do need a good mat. Try one of the various closed-cell Airex mats made by Torin. They offer the advantage of firmness and cushioning. These range from $50 to $150, depending on size and thickness. You also need good instruction. We recommend the book *Stretching* by Bob Anderson.

THE $5,000 VERSION

Strength equipment—$1,000 to $3,500. A good multistation gym provides the safest way to do full-body strength training and muscle toning when you're working out alone. These units will remind you of the old Universal weight machines from high school, except most of today's home versions are much more compact. The major improvement on the multigyms of recent years is the "no-cable-change" feature, which allows you to switch from one station to the next without the hassle of hooking and unhooking cables. It's very useful.

Multigyms generally have one or two weight stacks. Adding the second stack gives you extra stations, allowing for more than one user at a time. Single-stack units usually take up about 15 square feet of floor space, and two-stack machines require more than twice that much. If you're trying to conserve space, look for units with a vertical (rather than the standard flat) bench press. The only drawback to this style bench press is that it requires the less-comfortable standing leg curl.

• •

TRY IT BEFORE YOU BUY IT

The best all-around advice: Give exercise equipment a thorough test drive before you make the purchase. You can uncover unwanted quirks and shortcomings before you've plunked down the money and carted the unit home. Here are some shopping guidelines from Jon Valles, owner of Total Fitness Systems, a small chain of specialty fitness stores:

■ Inspect floor models. These often get a good amount of abuse from curious customers and are good indicators of how well the equipment will hold up at home with regular use.

■ Make sure you're comfortable on the machine in each position you'll assume during a workout.

■ Check to see if the machine is quiet when in use. On multigyms, make sure the cables and pulleys move smoothly and quietly.

■ Be sure that seats and pads are constructed with thick foam cushioning and durable upholstery and can be adjusted easily to fit your body.

■ Try out the electronics. Do they give you the feedback you want on calorie expenditure, speed, distance, and elapsed time? Are the controls understandable and easy to operate?

■ If you're on a budget, don't pay extra for chrome weight stacks. Although they look great, they don't give you a better workout, and they do require more maintenance.

■ Look for equipment that has at least a one-year parts/90-day labor warranty.

• •

Important stations to look for are a shoulder press, butterfly or pec deck, lat pulldown, low pulley for rowing and curls, and a leg extension/leg curl. The vertical knee raise, dip station, leg press, and stomach-crunch options are also worth considering.

For $1,000, the Newport gym by Pacific Fitness is a well-designed single-stack machine. Vectra, Hoist, Maximus, and Paramount also make good ones ranging in price from $1,000 to $3,000, depending on options. If you've got the budget, Pacific's Malibu gym ($3,500), complete with a seated leg press and calf-extension feature, is considered by many to be the best value for a two-stack machine.

Cardiovascular fitness—$1,500 to $2,600. The most popular choice for a high-end aerobic machine is a motorized treadmill. A good treadmill will have at least a 1½ horsepower motor, manual or motorized elevation (to simulate hills), sturdy handrails, and electronic feedback. (Stay away from units with built-in ear-mounted pulse meters; these meters are known to be inaccurate, and their presence indicates an inferior unit.) You'll spend around $1,500 for a good, basic treadmill. The Precor M9.1 is a sound investment at $2,000. Bodyguard, Aerobics, Inc. (PaceMaster), and Tunturi also make fine treadmills ranging in price from $1,500 to $2,500.

If there's extra money and space left over, a second or maybe even third cardiovascular machine is a good idea for the sake of beating boredom and doing cross-training. Some great choices:

■ Combination bikes. The CombiCycle EX80 (about $1,100) is a deluxe bike with a built-in pulse monitor that automatically adjusts resistance to maintain target heart rate. An additional $400 buys you a special seat attachment that converts the standard upright bike into a recumbent cycle, making it two bikes in one.

■ Dual-action climbers, as their name implies, give you a two-way workout, with arm levers that pump up your upper body as you climb. You'll find good-quality climbers for about $500 to $700 from companies like Precor and Tunturi.

■ Downhill-ski simulators can prepare you for the slopes while giving you a fun, vigorous aerobic workout. Scientific Sports Systems makes a unit called the Skier's Edge for $595, and Tunturi offers the SkiFit S530 for about $700.

The bottom line is that any good free-weight system or multigym can effectively improve your strength and body tone. And all well-made aerobic equipment is bound to improve your cardiovascular health. On the other hand, none of it will do a bit of good unless you use it. As sportscaster Roy Firestone once put it: "Unless you use your equipment regularly, you'll just have the fanciest digital clothes hanger on the block."

—Patrick Netter and Keri Casady

Even Though the Sound of It Is Something Quite Atrocious

Super calisthenics aren't so awful.
Jumping jacks, push-ups, and crunches
are coming back.

••••••••••••••••••••

"JUMPING JACKS, *readyyyyy . . . begin! One, two, three, four . . . one, two, three, four. . . . All right, hit the deck for some push-ups. I want those backs straight. Readyyyyy . . . one, two, one, two, one, two, one . . . hey, you, Goldilocks, keep that butt down! Okay, everybody, on your feet for squat thrusts. Readyyyy. . . ."*

For most of us, this is how it all began. It wasn't called training then, or working out, or (God forbid) aerobics. And you didn't wear Lycra or Gore-Tex or $75 sneakers when you did it. No, this was exercise in its purest form: calisthenics, the primordial exercise ooze from which we all sprang, clutching our sides, gasping for breath, and badgered by a guy wearing a whistle around his neck and a sneer on his face.

Done any calisthenics lately? We didn't think so. Nobody likes being forced to do something. It leaves a bad taste, like those stewed prunes they used to serve in the school cafeteria. Besides, as John Poteet, Ed.D., of the Institute for Aerobics Research in Dallas notes, with old-style calisthenics, "seldom was there an emphasis on technique, and you did so many repetitions, you felt like you had to hurt yourself to get fit."

But maybe it's time you give them another shot. Bad memories and bad form aside, calisthenics are efficient exercises. According to Gwen Robbins, a Ball State University physical education professor, you can burn up to 10 percent more calories by doing calisthenics than by running or walking for the same length of time. For the average man, that's about 110 calories for 10 minutes of jumping jacks or squats.

A WONDER WORKOUT?

Consider a calisthenics program as an adjunct to your other activities, whether you're into pumping iron or logging miles. "I use calisthenics as a substitute workout when I travel," says Robert

Morea, a former Mr. Delaware and now a triathlete and exercise physiologist. "They're also a good way to elevate the heart rate before lifting weights. They're good for runners, too, because they strengthen the upper body and abdominal muscles—muscles which are sometimes weaker in runners."

Coaches today know more about the right and wrong way to do these exercises, so injuries aren't as much of a problem anymore. If they were, trainers like Larry Starr of the Cincinnati Reds wouldn't be so hot on them. "There isn't one kind of exercise that can do it all," he says, "but calisthenics come close."

Long a part of the Reds' spring-training regimen, calisthenics have begun stretching into their regular season and off-season workouts over the past three years. The exercises cover four bases for the club: preactivity warm-up, postactivity cool-down, and improvement of flexibility and muscle tone. "We used to have players walking on the field 15 seconds before batting practice," Starr says. "Now the rule is that you warm up for 10 minutes with calisthenics before you hit."

When the season is over, Starr gives every player a one-sheet workout program to follow on the banquet circuit. We've adapted and supplemented his "hotel workout" with input from other experts to come up with an anytime, anyplace regimen.

• •

Have One for the Road

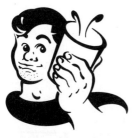

Endurance athletes commonly find that quenching their thirst during or after a long workout leads to an upset stomach. Especially in long runs in hot weather, downing that much-needed beverage when your throat is parched can seem to create more problems than it solves. Now, a Dutch study puts blame for the upset stomach on the dehydration, not the drinking. In experiments, athletes who kept well hydrated during extended workouts experienced no gastrointestinal distress. Those who didn't had stomach trouble when they drank following the workout. The researchers' conclusion: "Drink early on during a potentially dehydrating exercise bout, before a state of dehydration is reached."

You can use it as a warm-up to other activities. Or if calisthenics really are your calling, make it your entire program by building in aerobic training value. That means keeping your heart rate within 60 to 80 percent of your maximum rate (calculated by subtracting your age from 220) for a minimum of 15 to 20 minutes, three or four times a week. Bear in mind that while doing these exercises non-stop will maximize their aerobic value, it's okay to slow down during the transition from one exercise to another.

SAFETY FIRST

It's also wise to ease into things at the start, no matter what shape you're in. Most exercise injuries occur as a result of excessive repetitions. If you're a beginner, start with less than what's recommended here. And at any point, if something hurts, stop.

You'll notice some of the golden oldies of calisthenics, like squat thrusts and toe touches, are omitted from this list. That's because they could strain the lower back muscles.

Jumping jacks. Start with 3 minutes of these to break into a sweat and elevate your heart rate. They're a high-impact exercise, however, so do them on a soft surface like a mat, carpet, or grass.

Sprinter's run. Assume the position of a sprinter at the starting line, keeping your arms straight and your hands on the floor. Move your legs, one at a time, up to your chest in a simulated running movement. Try it for 30 seconds to 2 minutes, but remember to

• •

Wet Warm-Up

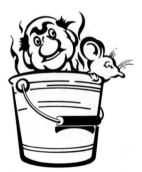

So you say you hate to waste time warming up before exercise? Researchers have found that using external heat sources may help prevent muscle injury. They reached this conclusion after warming the leg muscles of lab animals in saline baths and finding them more flexible than when cold. The study cautions that you shouldn't *replace* your active warm-up with a passive one, though it says passive warming could offer some additional protection.

keep your back straight and not lock your arms. That puts extra pressure on the joints.

Half squats. Another name for these could be not-so-deep knee bends. Plant your feet shoulder-width apart. Holding your head and back straight and keeping your feet and lower legs in straight alignment with your knees, squat until your thighs are parallel to the floor. Don't squat lower than that: Deeper bends can stretch knee ligaments, irritate the membranes surrounding the knee joint, and possibly damage cartilage. Contract your abdominal muscles as you come back up, and let your legs, not your back, do the work. Do 10 to 15 to start.

Push-ups. You may hear the coach's voice telling you to keep your butt down, but it's better to think in terms of not arching your back one way or the other; pretend you're in a body cast. Look downward and lower your body to the point where your elbows form a right angle. Try for ten.

Crunches. Strong abdominal muscles can prevent about 75 percent of all lower back problems. Yet according to Seattle kinesiologist Karen Clippinger-Robertson, the abs are active for only about a third of the time during full straight-leg sit-ups.

The solution: crunches. Your abs will be at work more than 95 percent of the time. Lie down and keep your lower back pressed to the floor. With your knees bent, feet on the floor, and arms crossed across your chest, lift up your shoulders slowly and gradually. Keep your chin tucked into your chest, and make sure your shoulder blades, not your head, touch the floor. Try for 12 to 15.

Running in place. Don't shuffle; keep those knees up. If you're a beginner, start with 15 seconds and work toward 3 to 5 minutes. To make sure you're not overdoing it, try the "talk test." If you can speak in a normal voice without gasping for breath, you're okay. If not, try a light jog or marching or walking in place.

Another option if running in place—or jumping jacks—bothers your ankles or shins: Step up and down on the first step of your stairs. Start with 15 seconds.

Stretching. A cool-down after your calisthenics will loosen you up so you won't wake up tomorrow feeling like you've been through the obstacle course at Quantico. But remember, don't bounce during any stretching exercise. A stretch should be *held* for 20 to 30 seconds and repeated three to five times. It should never hurt.

—John Hanc

Step Up in Life

*There must be a reason stair-climbing
machines continue to climb in popularity.
Here it is: You can burn 2,000 calories
in three 30-minute workouts a week.*

••••••••••••••••••••

STAIR-CLIMBING machines have ascended in popularity so
quickly that even though they've only been widely available for
about a year, they already rank as the most-used type of exercise
equipment in U.S. health clubs. Their fast rise to fame is probably
due to the fast results they bring: Three 30-minute workouts a week
on a "stepper" can burn up *2,000* calories. That regimen—along
with cutting out 1 tablespoon of butter a day and trading in a daily
glass of whole milk for a glass of low-fat—could help you shed a
pound a week.

Moving your legs up and down on the steps pits muscles
against resistance created by pistons, shock absorbers, or some
other sort of adjustable mechanical linkage. The machines are great
for developing the calves, thighs, and buttocks, and you get a good
cardiovascular workout in the bargain. Models with movable handles also help condition your upper body.

Stepping is low-impact exercise compared to running. And the
risk of muscle strain is much less than in weight training, says

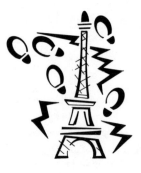

Bird's-Eye View

Want to visualize actually going
somewhere while you're on a stair
climber? These calculations from
the American Institute for Preventive Medicine may help: 16 minutes (at one step per second)
equals climbing the Washington
Monument; 28 minutes, the Eiffel
Tower; 36 minutes, the Empire
State Building. And if you're really
ambitious, go for Mount Everest—
14 hours.

Patrick Netter, a Los Angeles fitness consultant and author of the book *High-Tech Fitness:* "Stepping is less explosive, more controlled and rhythmical." It's also a good move for guys who get saddle soreness or lower back pain from riding a stationary bike, says Netter.

You can buy low-end models for less than $200 or pay ten times that for a top-of-the-line climber. Most machines are computerized. Very sophisticated units let you program different warm-up, workout, and cool-down sessions.

You may not need a $2,000 climber, but don't aim too low, warns Netter: "Low-end steppers are like low-end stationary bikes: They're unstable and noisy." He also likes models with at least some electronics. "Computerization provides instantaneous feedback, which can help motivate you," Netter says.

Among Netter's picks is the midpriced Precor 7.4: "It's almost as smooth as a $2,500 unit and has some of the same electronics, but costs under $900." Whatever type you use, follow these steps for maximum results:

■ Hold the handrails for balance only. The weight's got to be on your legs to guarantee the maximum burn. If you have to hang on to keep the pace, you're going too fast.

■ Make sure your knees move forward, staying over your toes. If you place your foot ahead of your knee and then try to lift up on that foot, your knee could get strained. Stair climbing isn't hazardous to knees when done properly. However, if you have an existing knee injury, you probably should stay off climbers and get your exercise by walking. Check with your doctor.

■ On programmable models, customize your workout time. You aren't stuck with the workout the computer has programmed (usually 15 minutes). If you want to go to 20 minutes, check your owner's manual or ask your health-club trainer for programming instructions.

■ Be specific. To tone buttocks muscles, take higher steps, letting the machine carry your foot farther down. To work the abdominals, take shorter steps, keeping your feet a little forward of your upper torso.

■ Put the machine in a cool spot in your home. A room comfortable for couch reclining may seem like a sauna while you're step inclining. And despite the obvious jokes about "Stairway to Heaven," rock music isn't the best accompaniment to your workout. The beat is too dominant, which can throw off your pacing. Show tunes or classical music are better choices.

If you buy a stair climber, will you use it or will it become another expensive rack to throw your clothes on when you get home from work? Netter says despite the intensity of the exercise, there's a high adherence to stair climbing compared with rowing and riding stationary bikes. "It could be the rhythmic nature of the workout," he says. "You go into almost a meditative state."

—Gloria McVeigh

Workout Tips from the Pros

These guys know how to exercise efficiently and safely. Take a few hints from Pat Croce, physical conditioning coach for the Philadelphia Flyers and 76ers, and others.

• • • • • • • • • • • • • • • • • • • •

NOT EVERY GUY HAS the time, money, or temperament to hire a personal trainer. But probably just about everyone who exercises or plays a sport could use the advice of a trainer on how to get stronger, faster, and fitter without getting hurt.

Men's Health can't send a professional trainer to your gym to fit you with a tailored program, but here's some good advice from ten of the country's top pros.

PAT CROCE
PHYSICAL CONDITIONING COACH,
PHILADELPHIA FLYERS AND 76ERS

Get your heart into it. "Commit 2 hours a week to cardiovascular training. That's 30 minutes, four times a week. Build up to that—on the stationary bike, jumping rope, stair climbing, jogging. Be sure to stretch out and cool down. Supplement that with your secondary objective, strength training. Every guy should realize he has to fine-tune the anatomical braces he was born with: his muscles."

Stomach it. "Do trunk-strengthening exercises to strengthen the abdominal wall. It can help prevent back pain."

Croce recommends:

1. Crunches for the abdominals. "Keep your knees bent, feet flat, hands interlocked behind your neck or crossed and resting on your shoulders. While tightening your stomach, lift your shoulder blades off the floor no more than 30 degrees."

2. Reverse sit-ups for the abdominals. "Start with the same position, but keep your elbows flat on the floor. Lift your knees up to your chest and then lower them."

3. Bicycles for the obliques. "Again, keep your hands interlocked behind your neck or crossed and resting on your shoulders. Bring your elbow to touch the opposing knee, but bring your knee up to meet the elbow as well—like pedaling a bike."

4. Russian twists for overall trunk and abdominal strengthening. "This is an advanced exercise. Lie on your back with your arms flat on the ground, perpendicular to your trunk. Bend your hips at a 90-degree angle and point your toes to the ceiling. Bring both legs down together and touch your left hand. Bring both legs back to the vertical, then down to touch your right hand.

· ·

Don't Mess with Excess

Too many good athletes are ruined by overtraining, says David Costill, Ph.D., director of the Human Performance Laboratory at Ball State University in Muncie, Indiana. Distance runners and swimmers, he says, are the most prone to mileage obsession and therefore suffer the most overuse injuries. "There's a point of diminishing returns," Dr. Costill says in _The Physician and Sportsmedicine,_ "where athletes can do more work and gain nothing from it." You know you're overtraining when (1) you always feel "heavy" during exercise, (2) you have difficulty falling and staying asleep, and (3) your resting heart rate is elevated.

"Do each exercise in succession, and never do them two days in a row. Start with 10 of each, but maybe fewer of the Russian twist, and build up to 30 reps."

Think pizza. "Nutrition will be the most important facet of conditioning during this decade. I recommend you look at the day's allotment of calories as a pizza pie. Three-fifths—60 percent minimum—should be complex carbohydrates, then one-fifth protein and one-fifth fat."

KEOKI KAMAU
HEAD TRAINER, NFL SAN DIEGO CHARGERS

Get wet. "I tell athletes to drink eight 12-ounce glasses of water a day. I can't stress enough the importance of hydration. There's a simple test to see if you're hydrated enough for an athletic competition: If you're urinating regularly just beforehand, then you're ready to go.

"As for the Chargers, we want to make sure every player drinks a half-gallon of fluids through the course of a game. We have 45 players, and on any given game day, we go through 55 gallons of liquids."

While it's common sense to drink lots of fluids when you're exercising or playing in the heat, some guys don't know they also need to drink up when it's cold—say, if they're out running or cycling. As Kamau says, "Just because you're not sweating heavily doesn't mean you're not dehydrating. We played the Redskins once in cold weather, and players kept coming up with cramps. That was my fault because I should have made sure they started building up their hydration a few days before the game. Because of the cold weather, they didn't think it was necessary, and they suffered for it."

DAVE WOHL
ASSISTANT COACH, NBA MIAMI HEAT;
FORMER HEAD COACH, NEW JERSEY NETS

Pool your resources. "Ron Culp, the trainer for the Heat, and I work out on the road. We find that even if the hotel gym is limited, we can still get a good overall workout in the pool." Here's their regimen:

1. Sit-ups. "Stand facing the side of the pool and sink down in the water. Let your legs go limp and float a bit behind you. Extend your arms and grasp the pool's ledge. Pull with your abdominal muscles and lift up your legs until your feet touch the side of the pool right between your hands. Concentrate on only using the abdominals, then push and let your legs go back behind you. Repeat 15 to 20 times."

2. Side stretch. "Lift your leg to one side, all the way out of the water, then return. Also do the lifts frontward and backward. Alternate legs and do 10 to 15 reps on each leg."

3. Arm lifts. "Use the same motion you would for normal arm weight lifts, but open your palms and fingers to create more resistance in the water. Do 15 reps."

4. Jogging. "Tread slowly and stretch your limbs through their full range of motion. Don't let your feet touch the bottom of the pool—let the water's buoyancy keep you afloat. You won't need a large pool: 10 yards in length is enough. The resistance should raise your heart rate to its maximum aerobic range in 4 to 5 minutes. Continue for 15 to 20 minutes."

Elevate yourself. "Sometimes, instead of working out in the pool, I'll put on my Walkman and walk the stairs from the ground floor to the top and back. Sometimes I'll jog it, and either way I'll vary my steps—one or two at a time. Try to go for 25 or 30 minutes for the best benefit."

If you do this, keep your personal stereo on low volume; according to at least one audiologist, exercise paired with loud noise may make you more susceptible to hearing loss than loud noise alone. Also, if you're overweight, stair climbing may be too hard on your knees.

GENE MONAHAN
HEAD TRAINER, NEW YORK YANKEES

Remember the code. For a good diet, Monahan suggests in *The Professional Baseball Trainer's Fitness Book*, remember the code 4–4–4–3–2. "This reminds you to eat every day the prescribed servings of the five basic food groups. Specifically, fruits, vegetables, and grains should be taken in four servings a day (4–4–4); protein (through fish, poultry, nuts, and lean red meat), three servings a day (3); and milk and dairy products, twice (2)."

FRANCIS FELD
ATHLETIC TRAINER, PITTSBURGH STEELERS

Don't sacrifice your calves. "The calves and Achilles tendon are universal problem areas for anyone in my age bracket—I'm 35. I'm deathly afraid of blowing out an Achilles tendon. Anyone my age should be, especially if he's getting into racquet sports. To stretch my calves and Achilles tendon, I use a heel board, constructed of wood. It's set like an inclined ramp at a 30-degree angle. I'll stand on that for 3 or 4 minutes. I'll slowly lean forward until I touch the wall with my nose. Wear a watch and keep time, because it's easy to talk yourself out of staying in the stretch."

Perfect your style. "With free weights, I have younger guys and those with lifting-related injuries use just the bar for a while, so they can concentrate on technique.

"You should warm up before doing any lifting. I recommend a light jog of 300 to 400 yards to get your heart rate up. Be sure to stretch the muscle groups you'll be working. If you suffer from knee or lower back pain, avoid squats."

Feld's exercise for the triceps is challenging: "Lie flat on your back on a bench. Set the bar on the floor, and with your arms hanging behind your head, lift it up. Once you can do three sets of ten reps and there is no strain or pain the following day, you can move up in weight. Remember the emphasis is on motion. It should be smooth, slow, and deliberate, not jerking."

DON WINANT
EXERCISE PHYSIOLOGIST; MEMBER, TRIATHLON
FEDERATION MEDICAL COMMITTEE

Learn from the best. "Anyone who wants to train should see a sports medicine physician, exercise physiologist, or a coach with good credentials. You might as well start out right.

"Someone taking part in a new sport or training program tends to get excited about it and then overdo it. Another problem is that while people may know something about physiology, it's difficult to be objective. I was on the U.S. national swim team and have a master's degree in exercise physiology, yet I have a hard time being objective with my own training. A coach, on the other hand, can stand at a distance and look at you objectively—analyze your mechanics and technique."

Because triathletes are typically the independent type, they often fall into bad habits, Winant says. "Triathletes have to break the self-coaching trend, especially when it comes to swimming, which requires so much subtle technique. I'm a coached, competitive swimmer, and I've gone up against uncoached triathletes and taken 10 strokes for their 30."

Contact these groups for information about clubs, coaches, and masters programs in your area:

■ U.S. Cycling Federation, 1750 East Boulder Street, Colorado Springs, CO 80909; (719) 578-4581

■ U.S. Swimming, 1750 East Boulder Street, Colorado Springs, CO 80909; (719) 578-4578

■ U.S. Masters Swimming, 2 Peter Avenue, Rutland, MA 01543; (508) 886-6631

■ The Athletics Congress (running), Association Services, P.O. Box 120, Indianapolis, IN 46206

■ Triathlon Federation/USA, 1604 East Pikes Peak Avenue, Colorado Springs, CO 80909; (719) 630-2255

For a registry of local physicians and trainers specializing in sports medicine and sports performance, send $5 to The American College of Sports Medicine, Certification Department, P.O. Box 1440, Indianapolis, IN 46206; (317) 637-9200.

TIM NEAL
ASSOCIATE ATHLETIC TRAINER,
SYRACUSE UNIVERSITY MEN'S LACROSSE TEAM

No need to club yourself into shape. "Too many guys over 30 think they're going to get right in there and play recreational club sports. They think they're going to play their way into shape, and that's just not going to happen.

"Start off with aerobic work, at a low level but for at least 20 minutes a day. Start off at three times a week during the work week and once or twice on the weekend. Build yourself up to where you're going six days a week. Then lift weights to get some tone and develop some basic strength. Do that *before* taking up any recreational sport."

KEN KONTOR
EXECUTIVE DIRECTOR, NATIONAL STRENGTH
AND CONDITIONING ASSOCIATION

Ready, set goal. "Train for a set goal in athletics rather than for an obscure concept called fitness. As you train for your goal, you'll develop proper muscle balance, proper flexibility, the right amount of cardiovascular fitness. All of these factors will enable you to keep enhancing your level of performance. You'll be motivated because you're taking part in an activity you enjoy.

"Say you want to be a better tennis player, and there's a club tournament in six months. While you train for this goal, you'll work on strength training, develop aerobic fitness, work on tennis skills. You may also give up smoking to help you aerobically; you'll give up fatty foods in favor of carbohydrates because you need proper fuel; and because you're exercising to prevent injuries while you play tennis, you'll prevent injuries during your everyday activity."

**STEVE VICTORSON
CONDITIONING COACH, U.S. MEN'S SLALOM
AND GIANT SLALOM SKI TEAMS**

Carry your own gym. "The most important things for a skier are good abdominal and leg strength and leg-muscle endurance. Otherwise, you may get injured. To develop leg strength, in the off-season we focus on weight training and interval training. We limit distance work, because too much makes you skinny. We want to promote power and strength.

• •

End with a Bang

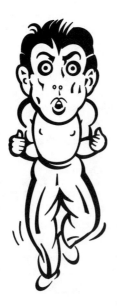

You can make your body produce steroidlike growth effects naturally, suggests new research at the University of Wisconsin. When athletes engaged in anaerobic exercises (short, high-intensity bursts of activity), their bodies produced twice as much human growth hormone as when they covered the same distance at a slower pace. For example, weight lifters who ended their sessions with a ¼-mile, all-out wind sprint might experience faster muscle growth and more rapid recovery between workouts, according to the study's leader. Human growth hormone, a powerful substance produced by the pituitary gland, is thought to help maintain muscle tone and burn fat.

"During the season, we have trouble finding workout facilities on the road, so we use a device called the Sport Cord for overall training. It's a piece of surgical tubing with handles at each end that provides resistance. It's like a mini-gym you can carry with you."

Several companies make surgical-tubing cords. The brand used by the U.S. Ski Team is not available in stores, but you can order color-coded cords of varying resistance directly from the company for $49 each (Sport Cord, Inc., P.O. Box 731004, South Lake Tahoe, CA 95731; 916-541-6961). The price includes shipping, instructions, attachments, and a travel bag. A set of videos demonstrating a complete training program is also available.

THOMAS W. HARRIS, M.D.
PHYSICIAN, U.S. SKI TEAM; AUTHOR OF *THE SPORTS MEDICINE GUIDE FOR THE EVERYDAY ATHLETE*

Eat right while working out. "If you have to eat just after or during heavy exercise, fruit or a complex carbohydrate like cereal usually works best. They digest easily and provide quick energy for working muscles."

—John Kirk

• •

Imagination Pays Off

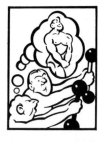

Visualization can help your sports performance, but you must picture yourself doing your best at the *specific* task you want to perform, suggests a study from the University of Newcastle in Australia. Two groups of men did as many sit-ups as they could within 30 seconds. After the first set, they were asked to "psych themselves up" in three different ways: by seeing, feeling, and experiencing their peak at doing sit-ups; by thinking of a situation that made them happy; or by counting backward from 500 by sevens. When the men did a second set, the ones who'd imagined doing sit-ups showed twice as much improvement as the happy fellows. The backward counters lagged way behind.

Part 10

TAKING CARE OF BUSINESS

Breaking Free

*How to jump-start a stalled career. Climbing the
corporate ladder is tougher than ever—
you need an edge.*

•••••••••••••••••••••

HE'S 41; HIS BOSS IS 33. He hasn't had a promotion in six years,
and he's beginning not to care anymore whether he's dressed for
success—or even whether his socks match. Meet a man standing
on a plateau, joined by a growing number of disillusioned middle
managers whose careers seem to have leveled off well short of the
executive suite.

Once upon a time, and not that long ago, the path to corporate
success was as automatic as an escalator. You got a good education,

started with a good company, and unless you had an affair with the boss's wife, you could expect to be promoted roughly every 12 to 18 months.

But no longer. Some corporate climbs are now about as negotiable as the north face of Everest, and the reason is simple: Not only do the paths to the summit have fewer handholds, but an unprecedented number of hands are reaching for them. Pressured to increase efficiency and profits in an ever-toughening global market, many companies started trimming their managerial ranks back in the early 1980s, and the cuts continue today. Accompanying those cuts has been a record number of 30- to 45-year-old baby boomers hitting what they thought would be their corporate stride. The result: a new upward immobility dubbed the "plateau effect"—a logjam of well-qualified would-be CEOs finding themselves stuck in the middle levels.

Things are expected to get worse before they get better. Managerial staffs are expected to be shaved by another two-thirds by the year 2000. What's a would-be VIP looking for his fair share of the good life to do?

Men's Health posed that question to some experts who keep their fingers on the pulse of such affairs, and it seems there may be some good answers after all for men whose careers have stalled.

SEEK THE JAGGED PATH

"There's a lot of talk about this plateau effect, and a lot of griping, but only because it's being looked at in the wrong way," says Greenville, South Carolina, career counselor Al Hafer. "There's more to life and more to a career than following an uninterrupted path upward."

Hafer coped with a plateau of his own as a 49-year-old middle manager at G.E. several years back. So he began studying for his master's degree in counseling—planning to use it to develop new capabilities at work. His job expanded, but he saw greater potential in working for himself. He took early retirement and started his own business in career counseling—simultaneously going for an Ed.D. Now he advises people on the very problem he solved. "I'm my own boss, and I feel I'm doing something that's important," he says. "I'm not going to say it was easy for all the years I had to attend classes at night while also working, but hard work was never what I was afraid of."

Nor was hard work the fear of Richard Geissler, who at the age of 32 found a way around the ceiling he hit in his career as a newspaper reporter. When he was bypassed for a position as city editor in favor of a 30-year-old newcomer, he asked to be transferred to his paper's state capital bureau and, before long, joined a senator's staff in Washington. At age 50, he's now a worldwide speaker for a major trade organization and feels that reaching a plateau may have been the best thing that ever happened to him: "It got my juices going. It made me look hard at my options. It got me thinking more creatively than I ever would have if I had stayed where I was."

It's not always a question of whether you should stay or leave, points out Henry de Montebello, 44, of the executive search firm Russell Reynolds Associates. Staying with your company but moving laterally can broaden your abilities, offer new challenges, and even help prepare you in the event a higher position should open up. "The executives who thrive in the future will be well rounded," says de Montebello. "You can't be a specialist at senior levels anymore; you have to be a generalist—someone who can see the big picture, a 'people person' who knows how to motivate."

David Hogberg, formerly of Quaker Oats, can vouch for that. By stepping laterally from manufacturing to product development and then to a post as a marketing manager, he not only avoided a plateau, he also gained the broad base of experience he would eventually need to win a top post. "My lateral moves were deliberate and they worked," he boasts at the relatively ripe age of 37. Today he's senior product manager at Con Agra.

Lateral mobility may indeed be the plateau antidote for many, experts say, especially if financial circumstances preclude a more entrepreneurial approach. Many large companies now are actually encouraging it, using internal job-posting systems as a way of helping employees out of the plateau trap.

ALL CAREERS ARE NOT CREATED EQUALLY

Some careers are more likely to stall than others. This advice may be a bit late if you've already started your boardroom climb, but experts warn you to beware of positions in purchasing, personnel, or data processing. The market for talent in these fields will stay level or shrink in the coming years, according to a business publication. Also steer clear of public relations (there's a big move toward doing corporate image work in-house), and avoid anything associated with the management of a company's real estate portfolio (especially while real estate remains soft). Accountants get regular pay raises but tend not to rise much in rank, and managers of all kinds who work overseas tend to forfeit the inside track to their brethren who stay close to the home office.

Other jobs are relatively immune to the plateau effect—in particular, law, medicine, education, and architecture. These fields offer more flexible forms of upward growth in companies that are less pyramid-shaped than most and a kind of job satisfaction that is less dependent on promotions.

Today more than ever, degrees count in the race to the top. The days of being able to rise like Horatio Alger from the mailroom to the boardroom are gone, a result of the trimming of middle-management positions that functioned as rungs for the upwardly mobile man. "On average, higher education equals higher pay," says Ken Hoyt, Ph.D., a Kansas State University career development specialist. More and more CEOs of the future are going to have degrees behind their names.

DO YOU REALLY WANT TO CLAW?

You also might want to ask yourself if the corporate climb is worth the effort for you. Clawing your way to the top is a lifestyle choice that involves much sacrifice. One 42-year-old manager at a steel extrusion plant in Illinois struggled for years to attain a top managerial post, only to find he didn't fit the mold once he got there. He hated dealing with the "people problems" his new post was responsible for. Ultimately, his frustration cost him his marriage, so he transferred to a small computer-software consulting firm where he could get his feet back on the ground. He has felt like a new man ever since. "I can smile again," he says.

Getting off the promotion path may not mean taking a financial beating. If you're good at your job, you'll get paid for it, says Columbia University business professor David Lewin, Ph.D. More and more companies are realizing the importance of keeping key people—even though they won't be able to promote them. Some firms have designed special tracks that offer independence and generous financial rewards—but may never lead to a title change. Given the choice, many men find it easy to sacrifice prestige for the satisfaction of having a life outside their career. "We may find ourselves moving back to a time when work wasn't such an exclusive source of gratification," says Beth King of the Center for Career and Life Planning at New York University.

Society still places great value on reaching the top of the heap, and it's risky to go against the grain. But if anyone can succeed in defying the standard, it's the members of the current generation. As one corporate consultant observes, "The baby boomers place creativity and self-expression at the center of their being."

"People who went through the Great Depression could resign themselves to finishing out their careers on a down note, but baby boomers are more willing to take chances because they expect more from life," says Al Hafer.

But maybe IBM physicist Philip Seiden puts it best. "If you haven't made it in society's eyes, who cares?" asks the 56-year-old Seiden, who withdrew from a senior management position 15 years ago to concentrate on research. "Have you made it in *your* eyes? That's what really matters. If you're happy, why strive for more? To satisfy your mother-in-law?"

—*Ron Heitzgebot*

Monday, Monday

*Could you use a few mental tricks to help
get you in gear on Monday mornings?
Brain research is pointing away from the
hot morning shower and toward visualization.*

•••••••••••••••••••••

YOU START MONDAY morning in a fog, locking your keys in the car, miscalculating the first transaction of the day, and spilling coffee on your supervisor's new Gucci briefcase. On top of it all, you feel like death warmed over. Buddy, it sounds like you've fallen victim to Sudden Shift Shock, the trauma caused by reentering the left-brained work world after a right-brained weekend.

Brain research has found that the two sides of the brain have very different functions. The left side handles logical, mathematical, and verbal tasks, while the right performs creative, spontaneous, intuitive, and emotional activities. So when you've spent the weekend indulging your right brain in pursuits like hot-tubbing, gardening, watching the tube, and skiing, it is often difficult to shift on Monday morning to the left-brained tasks that are required at most jobs.

It's a little bit like what happens when you're awakened by a phone call in the middle of the night and find you can't talk coherently. During sleep, your left brain is relatively inactive, and since verbalizing is performed by the left hemisphere, talking while in the right is difficult.

To avoid Sudden Shift Shock, you need to gently ease your brain from right to left on Monday morning by adjusting the way you awaken, bathe, dress, and get to work. Here's how.

Move slow, think fast. When the alarm goes off, form a mental picture of yourself leaping energetically out of bed, even if you're actually moving in slo-mo. This visual, which is very easy to muster while you're rousing from sleep, will give you some impetus to move.

As you leave the comfort of your bed, visualize yourself looking alert and admired in your office an hour and a half from now. This first step uses right-brained visuals to begin the shift to left.

Say something simple. Now you're ready for some left-brained verbalizing: On the way to the shower, say your name and address aloud, along with any other numbers or facts that are easily accessed.

• •

Execs with Pecs

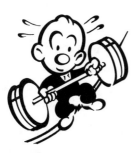

How do corporate honchos spell stress relief? E-X-E-R-C-I-S-E. Two-thirds of the 3,000 executives surveyed by James Rippe, M.D., of the University of Massachusetts Medical Center, say they exercise regularly—and nearly one-half say they do it to relieve stress. Their favorite activities? Calisthenics, running, fitness walking, stationary cycling, and weight lifting, in that order.

Don't stay near the water. Avoid baths or long, hot showers on Monday mornings. These encourage the right-brain daydreaming that quite naturally occurs when you're near water. Instead, take a left-brained power shower. Before you step in, assign yourself one work-related idea to focus on. Planning the first 15 minutes of your day is a good one. It will help you dredge up the unfinished business of Friday afternoon and get you on course for the day's work. Keep the water on the cool side so you won't be tempted to dally. Just get in and out, rubbing your face and hair briskly afterward.

Shift gears while commuting. The time you spend commuting to work offers a last opportunity to warm up your left brain. If you drive, you can preview your day's schedule and then focus your attention on your first or most troublesome project.

However, even the most disciplined thinker will find that the monotony of a long drive puts the left brain on hold. If you've been diligent about the previous mental exercises, you can utilize some moves to the right for developing innovative solutions to a work problem. Just don't forget to rein in your galloping imagination occasionally and apply it to practical situations.

If you ride the train or bus, it's often more difficult to control meanderings to the right because you don't have to stay alert to traffic or plan where you're going to park. But you are able to write and read. Reading quickly through your calendar or a job-related article or outlining a report you're going to write will ensure that you are "properly left" by the time you arrive at work.

—*Priscilla Donovan*

Corporate Blunders

Nine ways to assure yourself of failure. Here's an executive's guide to slipping up (and how to avoid it).

• • • • • • • • • • • • • • • • • • • •

STEP INTO ANY MALL bookstore and you'll find a dozen volumes on how to achieve nearly supernatural success at work. Donald Trump, Lee Iacocca, the guy with the weird hair who bought the shaver company—they've all been more than happy to share their secrets on how to make the big coin.

But where are the books for the man who wants to flee from success, who longs to *fail?* Why isn't there a manual of reverse alchemy for guys who desire to turn their gold medals into lead? Apparently there's a big audience waiting out there.

"Fear of success is common," says Mortimer Feinberg, Ph.D., chairman of BFS Psychological Associates, a New York management consulting firm. "It's the desire to get away from the pressures of achievement. Each new success is seen by some men as a new enslavement. One way to bail out of the increased responsibilities is to fail."

Other men, he says, feel unworthy of good fortune. They regard themselves as losers and look for ways to prove it. Hand one of them the reins and he'll strive to wrap them around his neck. "When people with low self-esteem succeed, they feel like frauds, so they sabotage their success," Dr. Feinberg explains. "Their policy is: It's better to sit in the back of the room and be discovered than to sit at the front of the room and be found out."

If you have a subtle urge to fail because of an aversion to responsibility or anemic self-esteem, Dr. Feinberg has done your homework for you. He interviewed a dozen top executives who were willing to share, anonymously, the secrets of their major screw-ups. *Now these proven failure techniques can be yours!* Consider them ammunition for shooting yourself in the foot. Of course, if failure is *not* what you have in mind, this guide can serve as a rundown of behaviors to resist.

Refuse to share your power. Insist on exclusive control and don't bother to solicit opinions, so that any flops are entirely to your discredit. "You won't survive long as an autocrat," Dr. Feinberg says. He cites the blunder of a young executive in a food-distributing company who was so enamored of a new yogurt-and-nut product that he didn't consult his sales staff before ordering boxcar-loads. Then he discovered his salespeople hated the stuff and would have gladly told him so if he'd asked. "He and his family were eating the yogurt for years," Dr. Feinberg says.

The converse of this is the survival strategy of David Dubinsky, the former head of the International Ladies' Garment Workers Union. "When things go right, I make the decisions," Dubinsky said. "When things go wrong, I look for a partner."

Organize the opposition. When you beat out a colleague for a promotion, make sure he stays an opponent. If you lose, hold a grudge. Never join forces with your rivals.

Lyndon Johnson was savvy enough to avoid this blunder, says Dr. Feinberg. "If he lost to an adversary, he sought reconciliation. That's why after challenging Kennedy for the presidential nomination, he could take second place on the ticket and go on to become president himself. And whenever he won, he was wise enough to bring the defeated rival into camp. He once said of J. Edgar Hoover, a potential adversary, 'I'd rather have him inside the tent pissing out than outside the tent pissing in.' "

Or as former baseball manager Leo Durocher once said, "I never let the four guys who hate me get together with the five who are undecided."

Be arrogant and treat your staff like hired hands. You'll quickly demotivate people, cripple their effectiveness, and turn potential friends into enemies. "Charles Revson of Revlon had a deserved reputation for a dictatorial attitude," says Dr. Feinberg. "He had a large security staff because he was afraid competitors would find a way to steal his product secrets. One time, a new security guard asked him for his pass and he instantly fired her. He said, 'She should have known who I am.' "

Adds Dr. Feinberg: "One of the executives at Estée Lauder claimed he staffed the Lauder company with refugees. 'From Germany?' someone asked. 'No, from Revlon,' he said."

Once you've made it to the top, disregard the people who put you there. Dr. Feinberg interviewed one executive with a strong record of achievements who tended to keep his board of directors waiting rather than interrupt his own tasks. His healthy bottom line didn't save him from getting booted in the end.

"Ignoring those who helped you rather than staying in loyal contact with them builds a lot of animosity," says Dr. Feinberg. "This turned out to be one of the most common errors of those who failed."

Defer all painful judgments regarding personnel. Wait until a disaster strikes to make the inevitable decision to fire that nice, incompetent person on your staff.

Take big financial risks for relatively small rewards. "When you get carried away by your own grandiosity, you forget the risk-to-reward ratio," says Dr. Feinberg. He gives the example of a manager who devotes a lot of his company's resources to cutting into a small, competitive market with a new product. "Even if the product succeeds, his company isn't going to make much, and if it flops, there's going to be a big loss."

Cling to a product or service beyond its heyday. Insist that your product, your baby, is immune to the market's life cycles. Dr. Feinberg points to the American autombile industry in the 1970s producing outmoded gas guzzlers while a squadron of Japanese compacts whizzed by in the fast lane.

Release a product or service before it's ready. If your idea is so hot it's practically radioactive, why let those drones in market research and production hold things up with their boring calculations? Go for broke—literally. One computer company announced an improved model prematurely, says Dr. Feinberg. Customers passed up the current version and waited for the better one. But the new model hit production snags and wasn't ready on time. Cash flow dribbled to a stop, and the company went belly-up.

Ignore your competitors. If your business is on a roll, don't keep looking over your shoulder at the other guys. You'll coast downhill. "The Swiss were shown some of the early digital watch designs, but they didn't want to make them. They said, 'It's not a watch—it doesn't have springs and gears.' They didn't think digital watches would put a dent in their market," says Dr. Feinberg.

By practicing even a few of these failure techniques, almost any executive can soon turn his throne of command into an ejection seat. Carefully avoid these pitfalls, and one day someone might ask you to write a book about how to get to the top.

—Peter Keely

How to Outwit a Rat

*Here are a few hints about dealing with the dirty play-
ers of office politics. Don't just get angry—get even!*

•••••••••••••••••••••••

PROBABLY ABOUT 80 percent of the guys at work are honest.
Another 15 percent are of questionable integrity. But face it, the
remaining 5 percent are out-and-out dirtballs, and if you're not careful, they'll get you.

How bad are these guys? Let's just say you wouldn't want one
to accompany your wife to that trade conference in Rio.

Men's Health has identified the various species of dirtballs who
inhabit the workplace. Here's a report on the five most common,
with useful tips on psyching each of them out.

Snidely Wite-Out. This character likes nothing better than to
take lengthy reports his subordinate has written, lather Wite-Out
over the poor guy's name, and then type in his own before passing
the work on to higher-ups.

Stealing credit for the labor of others is a common phe-
nomenon in corporate politics. And to a certain degree, you should
be proud when your superior depends on your fine work to advance
his cause. But Snidely's different. He'll steal your fire absolutely and
pass along none of the rewards. He'll tell his boss that it was he, not
some overworked underling, who came up with that novel way of
test-marketing toothpicks or tracking the motility of sperm. When
you've lost your due credit a couple of times, you have to start thinking about protection.

Solutions: First, document all your work, even if only in a personal journal that you can bring forward should somebody question
your contributions. Next, you have to learn to be more vocal about
your behind-the-scenes toilings. Consider sidling up to the big
boss at the company Christmas party and uttering the likes of
"How 'bout this crazy weather? By the way, has Snidely gotten
around to sending you my new proposal about doing a video on dog-
grooming tips?"

Of course, more direct action may be necessary. When someone turns to you in the elevator and says, "That Snidely's full of crazy

ideas. Did you hear his latest brainstorm about dog-grooming videos?" don't just stand there with your mouth hanging open. It's time to march into Snidely's office and demand to know what happened.

Moreover, when kudos are circulated following a successful project and you aren't even mentioned, don't hesitate to make a stink. Instead of wimpishly imploring Snidely, "Why wasn't I given any credit?" say, "I deserve credit on this. I was unfairly overlooked. You know this. I know this. Let's talk about ways of straightening this thing out."

Forgetful Freddie. This is the fellow who effusively praises a co-worker's presentation in a planning meeting, only to deny he ever supported it when the project flops.

Solutions: Immediately following the planning meeting, send Freddie a brief memo—some call it a "cover-your-ass" memo—in which you thank him for his support. Include specifics, such as: "I was particularly encouraged when you said my proposed strategy represented a brilliant new direction for our division."

If Freddie doesn't respond, it's tacit approval, explains Virginia E. Schein, Ph.D., a professor of management at Gettysburg College. Since Freddie's endorsement of the project is now on paper, he's unlikely to run to senior management to claim disapproval six months later.

Monty, the Phony Mentor. Monty promises his "protégé" unwavering support for a promotion that mysteriously winds up going to someone else. Instead of giving his protégé the avowed stellar recommendation, Monty secretly tells all concerned that the guy is a lazy lowlife who needs a bit more experience before he can advance. None of that's true, of course, but the mentor has grown to depend on the man's hard work. When the protégé asks why he wasn't promoted, Monty denies knowing the reason.

Solutions: When it comes to questions about career advancement, never settle for vague answers. If you're denied an expected promotion, do some serious digging to find out what went wrong. Pump potentially knowledgeable co-workers for information. Interview the person responsible for the decision and subtly drop the fact that good old Monty promised a favorable recommendation. Then, to force Monty's hand, ask to see a copy of the letter of recommendation, suggests Stuart Schmidt, Ph.D., chairman of the

Department of Human Resources Administration at Temple University. Be creative and delicate about how you broach the subject, though. For example, explain that the act of keeping the letter in your drawer and referring to it from time to time is something that motivates you to push harder in times of self-doubt.

Loose Lips Louie. This fellow never quite comes out and says, "Tell me all the intimate details of last night's sexual encounter with your secretary and her best friend." Or, "By the way, would you please explain your step-by-step strategy for taking over control of the purchasing department?" Instead, he lulls his victims into opening up to him by confiding some seemingly revealing, but in fact harmless, story about one of his own peccadilloes. Once he's got the goods on you, he has power, explains Washington, D.C.–based organizational psychologist Peter Wylie, Ph.D. You can be sure he'll break the confidence when it's to his advantage.

Solutions: The obvious course is to keep your lips sealed in this guy's presence. And once you have your eyes open to the problem, the Louies of the world are fairly easy to spot: "You can be pretty certain that someone who is always coming into your office with juicy bits of information about other people is not to be trusted," says Mardy Grothe, Ph.D., coauthor of the book *Problem Bosses.* "But it's hard to know when first meeting someone if they are the type to break a confidence."

To ensure that a new and unknown guy doesn't blab, work to achieve a point-system confidence equilibrium. If you divulge something, make sure you've learned something of equal value from the other guy. For example, let's say the secret "I'm planning on making a raid into the eastern region's turf " is worth about four points. You can safely drop this missile if Louie has divulged a four-pointer of his own, such as "I'm sleeping with the boss's girlfriend." Keep things even, and you'll be perfectly safe.

Spineless, the Rumor King. Unlike Louie, who deals in reality-based gossip, Spineless just makes it up as he goes along. Often the little poison darts he throws are shaped in the form of questions, such as "Is there any truth to the rumor that Jim in Management Information Services is in a drug detox clinic and not really on a fishing trip in British Columbia?"

Human nature being what it is, people within earshot will remember the phrase without the question mark. And when the boss just happens to hear concern from three or four independent sources about Jim's drug problem, he's likely to start thinking less favorably about poor old Jim.

Solutions: If you want to keep Spineless from starting rumors about you, you have to be highly alert. Chances are, he'll start with something milder than the above example. He might plant rumors that you are behind in meeting a particular deadline, for example. At the point where a few co-workers say, "Hey, I hear you're having trouble meeting that deadline," your antennae should twitch, and you should track the rumor to its source.

Then you confront the dirtball much the way you confronted the playground bully of your youth, with something on the order of "I know what you're saying. It has to stop. If you have a problem with me, you should deal with me directly."

By targeting the problem in such an up-front manner, you let Spineless know that you have his number. That can be very useful, as most weasels are good at knowing when to run for cover. Still, under no circumstances can you ever assume the battle with a guy like this is over. As Dr. Grothe points out, "You can't strike a good deal with a devious person. All deals are on soft ground."

If confrontation isn't working, fight fire with fire. Follow the advice of Jack Levin, Ph.D., a Northeastern University professor of sociology—and a student of gossip—who suggests getting the best-connected person in the company to spread a denial to the rumors.

And if all else fails, there's a fall-back position which has a lot of history behind it. In the words of Dick Munro, chairman of the executive committee of Time Warner, Inc.: "If you've got a guy who is really doing awfully bad stuff to you and nothing else works, maybe you just simply punch him." He adds, "I would suspect that's very high risk, by the way."

True. But isn't taking risks what they're paying you the big bucks for?

—David Diamond

Harvesting Harmony

"Executive counselors" are a new breed in the
corporate world. They're called in when big egos collide.

• • • • • • • • • • • • • • • • • • • •

SOMETIMES THE SMARTEST executives are no shrewder than
the rest of us when it comes to managing their own egos.

Take the case of executives David Hammer and Stanley Ham
(although their names *sound* like pseudonyms, they're real). A few
years ago, Hammer, the 36-year-old founder of a Virginia telemar-
keting company, was anguished that his most profitable branch
office was being managed by the 33-year-old Ham. Hammer felt that
Ham was rebellious, negative, and slow in seizing opportunities for
higher profits. "I thought he lacked the vitality, the enthusiasm, or
the oomph to come up with solutions to the business problems,"
Hammer remembers.

Ham had big problems with Hammer, too. The younger man
yearned for a fatherly mentor but instead saw his boss as a reincarnation of his worst high-school coach: dogmatic, insensitive, a one-
way communicator. "I was so angry at him I had to shadowbox with
one of those clown-face balloon bags so that I wouldn't resort to
actual violence," Ham says today. "Not that I was planning to hit
him, but I was harboring resentments that were that strong."

Ultimately, he got so fed up he resigned. Hammer, realizing
he'd be foolish to let his most productive manager walk, consulted
with his father, who sits on the company's board. The father
referred his son to David Charney, M.D., a psychiatrist specializing
in executive counseling. Dr. Charney met with the two antagonists
separately. "He could see that we were a lot alike," Hammer says.
"We just weren't hearing each other, and neither of us felt appreciated." Dr. Charney spotted Ham's resentment toward authority figures and suggested the men regard each other as coach and star
athlete. The three began meeting monthly.

"Eventually," Hammer says, "we dropped our guard and related to each other as human beings." "I've matured," Ham offers.
"I'm not as reliant on recognition. My work is its own reward."

WHEN EXECUTIVE EGOS COLLIDE

Across America, upper-management executives routinely bash heads like rams during mating season. Chairmen clash with CEOs, CEOs fight with presidents, vice presidents and partners trash each other. They wrangle over promotions, over turf, over the company's future, or just about personal style. Gossipy stories about their boardroom battles are standard fare in the business press.

But when these internecine wars lead to abrupt resignations or dismissals, when the people are too valuable to lose, some companies hire a psychologist or psychiatrist to mediate. What's most remarkable about this therapy isn't the treatment itself—it borrows the techniques of marriage counseling and applies a business twist. What's most unusual is the clients. Ordinarily, upper managers are the last to admit they need help of any kind, let alone psychological counseling. Yet a growing number of them are swallowing their pride and accepting help, for the sake of their companies if not for themselves. And in doing so, they're learning some lessons that all of us can profit from.

It isn't clear how many therapists practice in this field today. Because so many executives attach a stigma to psychotherapy, management psychologists are inclined to camouflage themselves. You don't call them "doctors"; you call them "executive counselors," "management consultants," or "communication specialists." Their suites don't have leather couches or framed portraits of Freud; they have that mahogany-desk, potted-plant, corner-office look of executive chambers.

Trappings aside, it works a lot like marriage counseling. The specialist starts by interviewing one client at a time—or both together to avoid the appearance of favoritism. He gains their trust, serves as a translator, assists in role playing, helps them act out confrontations, and becomes a model of empathy and openness. The first joint sessions tend to be a bit rocky. Pent-up anger is often unleashed early on.

"I was with two lawyers," recalls Wilbert R. Sykes, M.D., of TriSource Group, Inc., an executive counseling firm in New Rochelle, New York. "When I tried to paraphrase what one of them had said, I misstated his position. He yelled at me and said I was absolutely stupid. Then his partner turned to me and said, 'Now can you see what I'm going through?' "

IN MANY WAYS LIKE A MARRIAGE

In companies run by two partners, such marriagelike antipathy is very common. Dory Hollander, Ph.D., a St. Louis psychologist who specializes in management and careers, tells of two architects who built a thriving design firm in the Southwest. In midlife, one of them had become bored. He nodded off at meetings, regularly punched out early without an explanation, and sloughed a lot of work onto his increasingly resentful partner. "All of this had been swept under the rug," Dr. Hollander says. "There was no communication between them other than 'How are you?' 'Fine.' 'How do the books look today?' "

After months of depression and panic attacks, the disengaged partner phoned Dr. Hollander, then hemmed and hawed for weeks before telling her why he called. Here, counseling led to divorce rather than reconciliation: The man left the firm after realizing he was staying only for the money and prestige. "They went their separate ways," says Dr. Hollander, "but instead of a blowout and a law-

· ·

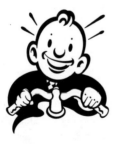

Get a Leg Up on Your Colleagues

More than three million Americans ride their bicycles to work. Here are three reasons bicycle commuting is good business:

■ A University of California study says commuting by car raises blood pressure, lowers frustration tolerance, and fosters negative moods. Conversely, cycling relaxes nerves, sharpens mental acuity, and bolsters your spirits.

■ Bike commuters get to work on time. More than half of commutes are 5 miles or less. Studies have shown that bikes can cover this distance as fast as cars or public transit. What's more, cyclists can slip through gridlock and circumvent traffic jams.

■ Biking saves money. You don't need gas. You don't need insurance. And a secure bike lock costs less than $100, compared to annual auto parking-space costs ranging from several hundred dollars to more than a thousand.

suit, the resolution was peaceful." Therapists say such depression and panic aren't uncommon symptoms of executive feuds; clients have shown up with everything from asthma to torticollis, a bizarre, paralyzing twist of the neck.

Ego, though, is what executive counseling is ultimately all about. Executives usually get where they are by being right a lot, and even when they're wrong, they're not inclined to admit it. Once they've taken a position, it's not easy to back down gracefully. Management consultants help these executives rein in their egos and teach them to respect and acknowledge another person's opinion.

"We try to take them from an egocentric point of view to a relativistic point of view," says Dr. Wilbert Sykes. "Getting people to appreciate what's going on from an objective rather than a subjective point of view is the most fundamental thing we do." Says San Francisco psychologist James Terrill, Ph.D., "You get them to see that the conflict doesn't have to be win/lose, that there can be a win/win resolution."

TOUGH GUYS IN SUITS

This need to win, therapists say, is true of men in general. "A skill that women are taught from the earliest years, and what men lose track of," says Dr. David Charney, "is empathizing with another person's point of view." Men, he says, need to find more empathy in themselves. Daniel Kegan, Ph.D., president of Elan Associates, a Chicago organizational development firm, puts it this way: "The traditional macho male finds it difficult to do things that will resolve conflict. It's not typical male behavior to say 'Gee, I'm sorry, I made a mistake.' "

Knowing that, the executive therapist speaks like a real guy. "While I wear the cap of a psychiatrist, I take it off as soon as possible," says Dr. Charney, who sometimes meets his clients over lunch. "I need them to understand that I'm talented in that area. But more so, I want them to see me as a businessman who understands their problems. I use business jargon instead of psychiatric jargon, and I keep up on what's going on in the business world. I want to keep it 'just us guys talking.' "

No one knows exactly how many executives are getting this sort of therapy, but the number seems to be growing. As for David Hammer and Stanley Ham, both are wiser and richer after ten months of sessions. When the emotional storm blew over, they saw their real business dilemma: Ham couldn't hire enough skilled sales-people on his budget. "The real problem was the shrinking labor force in Virginia," explains Hammer, who came up with the extra bucks and now credits the counseling with helping to boost his com-pany's annual sales from $2.7 million to $4 million in four years.

"A lot of executives see all this as a weakness," says Ham. "But obviously, they're wrong. Getting counseling can be a strength."

—Kerry Pechter

Part 11

HOT READING FROM TOP BOOKS

Men Need Men

In nearly every culture, "the lodge" has been associated with certain qualties of men being men together.

● ●

IN NEARLY EVERY culture, the lodge—as a mythic image, a metaphor, and often a physical place—has been associated with certain qualities of men being men together. In traditional cultures, the sweat lodge is where songs and prayers are offered all through the night. Other lodges, like my father's, feature the sounds of billiard balls and poker chips. When Ralph Cramden and Ed Norton or Stan Laurel and Oliver Hardy needed time to get themselves out of trouble, especially with their wives, they invariably headed for the lodge.

Although sweat lodges, Elks and Rotary gatherings, and men's rap groups don't serve precisely the same functions, they do tend to share some rather enduring ideas: Refuge. Sanctuary. Privacy. Friendship. Camaraderie. As a physical location, the lodge provides a retreat from concerns about money and work, family pressures, and responsibility.

And a place to get away from women. Not because women are the enemy, but because they are, in fact, women, and men are men. Contrary to the misguided assumption that the complete eradication of gender differences somehow adds up to equality, men and women continue occasionally to need time away from one another in the company of their own gender.

From *To Be a Man* by Sam Keen; edited by Keith Thompson

Rational about Money

There are "laws" of money.
Among them: Time is not money; time is time.

•••••••••••••••••••••

IT IS NOT LIKELY that any of us, no matter how hard we try, will ever be able to completely eradicate the Money Complex in ourselves. The way money both influences and reflects our life stories places a limit on the amount of financial objectivity we can achieve. But just because we may never behave like paragons of sanity when it comes to money doesn't mean we have to let it make us *insane*. And just because we can't operate with utter objectivity doesn't mean we can't operate with a healthy amount of decisiveness, flexibility, confidence, and competence.

It's difficult to conceive of many absolute truths about something so paradoxical as money. But many things are paradoxical, and still we find we do best if we devise a set of truths to live by and stick with them in the absence of anything better. The nature of the universe is a paradox, but we inhabit the earth and explore our solar system according to the laws of physics as we conceptualize them.

There are, in the same sense, "laws" of money, too:

■ Money is neither god nor devil.

■ Money can symbolize anything we wish it to.

■ Much of the way we behave toward money is unconsciously motivated.

■ Money is safest when it is "out of the closet," discussed calmly and candidly with one's spouse, one's parents, and, most especially, one's children.

■ A degree of detachment from money is desirable. A disdain for money is detrimental.

■ In order to have enough money so that one does not have to think about it, one must think about it.

■ Those who feel they don't deserve to have much money usually don't.

■ Where money is given there is expectation.

■ Where money is taken there is obligation.

■ Work goes better when money is a by-product *of* work and not the principal motivation *to* work.

■ We are not what we earn, owe, or own. We are what we are.

    And last:

■ Time is not money. Time is time.

From *If I Think about Money So Much, Why Can't I Figure It Out?* by Arlene Modica Matthews

Fatherly Ways

To men, children are a commitment,
an investment, an obligation, and a hope.

●●●●●●●●●●●●●●●●●●●●●

CHILDREN, FOR MEN, are a commitment, an investment, an obligation, a hope. They are men's chief contribution to the world and justification for their lives. The children are loved for themselves, yes, but they are also loved as carriers of their fathers' efforts and hopes and selves. The two kinds of love can't be disentangled.

It's easy to underestimate men's investment in their children. Men so often display that investment not by being present and nurturing but by working hard, somewhere else, to provide for the children. That the men believe their work is a way of caring for their children may be evident only through framed photographs on their desks, but in the backs of their minds, they value their work at least in part because it makes it possible for them to support their children.

Fortunate are men whose marriages have persisted and who have successfully launched their children into adult life. Thoughts of their children can then provide them with reassurance that whatever else happens in their lives or has happened, in this critical respect, they have done well.

From *Staying the Course* by Robert S. Weiss

Getting Even

*At a certain point,
there is a baffling stupidity to anger.*

• •

OF COURSE, REVENGE is frequently captious and childish. A drunk with a cleft palate was teased and mimicked by snowmobilers in a bar I occasionally visit. He demolished a dozen of their machines with his three-quarter-ton pickup. A friend in San Francisco was justifiably enraged by his landlord. He bored a hole in the roof and gave the landlord's apartment a several-thousand-gallon hosing that, unfortunately, streamed through the floor into his own apartment.

And at a certain point, there is a baffling stupidity to anger. Years ago, when I learned that my sister's first husband had slugged her, I made inquiries to find out how I could get him murdered; but

I was on a Guggenheim grant and could scarcely handle the seven-grand fee. I settled for a phone threat. Years before that, I set out to murder the drunken driver who had killed my father and sister; but he, too, had been killed in the accident. I suspect that affairs of the blood and those of love bring us closest to the flash point.

From *Just Before Dark* by Jim Harrison

In Earnest Pain

Hemingway's drinking wasn't his only problem.

• •

ERNEST HEMINGWAY'S ability to hold his liquor was remarkable. Lillian Ross, who wrote his profile for the *New Yorker,* does not seem to have noticed he was drunk a lot of the time he talked to her. Denis Zaphiro said of his last safari with Hemingway: "I suppose he was drunk the whole time but seldom showed it."

Hemingway also demonstrated an unusual ability to cut down his drinking or even to eliminate it altogether for brief periods, and this, in addition to his strong physique, enabled him to survive. But the effects of his chronic alcoholism were nonetheless inexorable. Drinking was also one of the factors in his extraordinary number of accidents.

The year 1918 saw him blown up in the war and smash his fist through a glass showcase. Two years later, he cut his feet walking on broken glass and started internal bleeding by falling on a boat cleat. He burned himself badly smashing up a water heater (1922), tore a foot ligament (1925), and had the pupil of his good eye cut by his son (1927). In spring 1928 came the first of his major drinking accidents when, returning home, he mistook the skylight cord for the lavatory chain and pulled the whole heavy glass structure down on his head, sustaining concussion and needing nine stitches. He tore his groin muscle (1929); damaged an index finger with a punch bag, was hurt by a bolting horse, and broke his arm in a car smash

(1930); shot himself in the leg while drunk and trying to gaff a shark (1935); broke his big toe kicking a locked gate, smashed his foot through a mirror, and damaged the pupil of his bad eye (1938); and got two more concussions in 1944, by driving his car into a water tank in the blackout and jumping a motorcycle into a ditch. In 1945, he insisted on taking over from the driver to take Mary to the Chicago airport, skidded, and hit a bank of earth, breaking three ribs and a knee and denting his forehead (Mary went through the windscreen). In 1949 he was badly clawed playing with a lion. In 1950 he fell on his boat, gashing his head and leg, severing an artery, and concussing himself for the fifth time. In 1953 he sprained his shoulder falling out of his car, and that winter, there was a series of accidents in Africa: bad burns while drunkenly trying to put out a bush fire, and two plane accidents, which produced yet another concussion, fractured skull, two cracked spinal discs, internal injuries, a ruptured liver, spleen, and kidneys, burns, a dislocated shoulder and arm, and paralyzed sphincter muscles. The accidents, which usually followed drinking, continued almost to his death; torn ligaments, sprained ankle climbing a fence (1958), another car crash (1959). On July 2, 1961, after various unsuccessful treatments for depression and paranoia, he got hold of his best English double-barrelled shotgun, put two canisters in it, and killed himself.

From *The Intellectuals* by Paul Johnson

Watching the Leaves Fall

Enjoying leisure must sometimes be learned.

•••••••••••••••••••••

MANY OF US WOULD hesitate to use the word *leisure* to describe what we do when we are not at work. After all, our prowess on the squash court, our meals at fancy restaurants, and our trips to resorts are all part of the professional success package. Rather than leisure, these activities are further proof of our overall accomplishments.

The notion of leisure, in fact, is likely to have negative connotations for those who have steadfastly pursued careers and ever-higher professional goals. A life of excessive leisure is a life that is unserious and unfocused. We equate leisure with idleness, uselessness, even boredom. We may even panic during those rare moments when we have time on our hands. It is as if, in the world beyond the cult of busyness, there lies a lonely abyss, filled with the endless buzz of daytime soap operas and Oprah Winfrey.

Work for many of us is an easy and acceptable way to fill the hours. In our professional lives we have clear rules to follow and goals to meet. By contrast, it is completely up to us to invent the success framework for our leisure. For many of the same reasons, however, that we have been unable to take control of our jobs, we have also found it difficult to take charge of our free time. Instead, whether we are watching television, dining out, or attending a sports event, we often end up being passive participants in our leisure lives.

Learning to be successful at free time first means accepting that having enough time after work to pursue activities that are productive and meaningful doesn't imply that we are losers. Setting limits in no way means signing your career death sentence. What it does mean is getting used to the idea of having more time for yourself, your family, and your community. Many of us recoil at the idea of leisure. Too much of it means we are weak, dull, losers. While we may yearn for the front porch and its promise of community and meaning, we feel it would be an unproductive waste of time to spend an evening or an afternoon sitting on that porch immersed in our thoughts and dreams; talking casually with our neighbors; watching the leaves fall and the sun set.

From *Downshifting: Reinventing Success on a Slower Track* by Amy Saltzman

Rules of the Road

*Never eat in any restaurant
with a king or a fox in the name.*

● ● ● ● ● ● ● ● ● ● ● ● ● ● ● ● ● ● ● ●

NEVER EAT IN ANY restaurant with kings, foxes, coaches, or horses in the name. Beware of the word *gourmet*. If a restaurant says it serves gourmet food, you are going to get a frozen dinner that has been warmed up in the microwave.

Never sleep on the side of the bed next to the telephone. That is where everybody else sleeps, for the convenience of answering the morning wake-up call, and that is where beefy traveling salesmen sit during the day to call their clients. The mattress on that side of the bed is always broken down, and you will find your slumber interrupted by the need to keep grasping the uphill sheet to keep from rolling off toward the telephone.

Carry a rubber sink-stopper in your pocket. The mechanical arrangements for keeping water in motel-room sinks never work.

Always ask for dry toast at breakfast, with butter on the side, so they do not slather that greasy stuff on your toast back in the kitchen. I don't know what it is, but it isn't butter.

Never be without a big safety pin. The curtains of motel-room windows never quite meet in the middle. They must be pinned unless you want a direct shaft of bright sunlight to fall across your eyes in the morning, an hour and a half before it's time to get up.

You could carry a knife, scissors, tweezers, magnifying glass, can opener, corkscrew, toothpick, awl, and Phillips screwdriver—or you could carry a Swiss Army knife. I find an essential use for mine nearly every day on the road.

Hotel-room radios never work. If you want a little news in the morning and a little Haydn at night, as I do, you should have a fifteen-band FM/long-wave/medium-wave/shortwave/alarm-clock Sony ICF-7700 in your bag. It's the size of a paperback book, weighs less than a pound, and is always there to keep you company.

If you must work at night, carry a 100-watt light bulb. Forty-watt bulbs are manufactured exclusively for the motel trade. They provide enough light to find your way to the bathroom but not enough to read by.

Whatever you order in a café, do not order chili. Café chili is invariably disappointing and potentially lethal.

Gift shops are well named. There's never anything in them that you would want to keep for yourself.

Gas station attendants become more polite the farther the gas station is located from the main highway.

From *A Life On the Road* by Charles Kuralt

Sound Advice

There are two questions a man must ask himself:
"Where am I going?" and "Who will go with me?"

• •

I HAD RECENTLY BEEN divorced after a 17-year marriage. My children were living a thousand miles away. I was madly in love with a beautiful young woman. She was rapidly slipping away from me, and I could already feel the other man lurking in the shadows. To protect myself against the coming loss, I had already provided myself with another lover to fill my empty hours and lonely nights.

My life was coming apart at the seams.

One day I went to talk with a friend of 25 years, grandson of a slave, philosopher, a man acquainted with darkness and the journey of the spirit. Through a long afternoon we talked and sipped bourbon. I told him about the pain of the divorce and my disintegrating romance.

The last thing he said before I left was probably the single most important bit of advice I ever got about being a man. "Sam," he said, "there are two questions a man must ask himself: The first is 'Where am I going?' and the second is 'Who will go with me?' If you ever get these questions in the wrong order, you are in trouble."

From *Fire in the Belly: On Being a Man* by Sam Keen

Special Treatment

*One of the oldest principles of
management is hogwash.*

• •

I THINK I STARTED maturing as a manager when I discovered that one of the oldest principles of organizational management
was hogwash. That principle is stated in many ways, but the military guys used to put it best: "Nobody gets special treatment
around here."

How many times have you been exposed to—or used—that old
management hiding place? In the military, they might also say,
"If we do this for you, Lieutenant Autry, we'll have to do it for
everyone."

I used to want to say, "No, sir, you could do it just for me."

What I realize now is that the professed aversion to special
treatment was all delusion anyway; people in every organization,
including the military, get special treatment all the time. Unfortunately, much of it has tilted toward "in" groups, such as West
Pointers or graduates of the right business school. That kind of
"special treatment" is favoritism and discrimination.

But there's another kind of special treatment that, simply
stated, is a manager's willingness to bend the rules to accommodate
every person's specialness, and this special treatment is an increasingly important tool in the workplace.

Some people do good work but are slow; some do fast work but
are sloppy. Some are morning people; some do better in the afternoon. Some have children who cause schedule problems; some
have elderly parents. Some need a lot of attention and affirmation;
some want to be left alone to do their work. Some respond more to
money, less to praise; some thrive on praise. Some are workaholics;
some work only for the livelihood. Then, of course, some are very
bright; some are slow. Some are men; some are women.

Who in the world could believe that all those special needs
could be accommodated without some special treatment?

I've made exceptions to corporate rules to help get an employee's family through overwhelming financial and emotional distress.

I've made similar exceptions for employees needing assistance to recover from substance abuse.

Our company has flex hours—a nice innovation, but even so, an individual employee may need to flex the hours a bit beyond the policy from time to time. My policy is that it's between the person and the supervisor, and the supervisors know that I generally choose the side of flexibility.

The road of special treatment is not without peril, and it makes day-to-day management much trickier and more time consuming. You must consider the impact on the group, the legal risks, and the questions of equity and justice, in addition to the record and commitment of the person involved. Then, if at all possible, decide in favor of special treatment.

There will be the potshotters and detractors, the people who worry about precedent and control, who worry that the other employees will become resentful.

But there is only one answer to that: Trust the great majority of your employees to know that you are trying to do the right thing and that their time will come.

When someone complains, just say, "Everyone gets special treatment around here."

From *Love and Profit* by James A. Autry

A (Very) Short History of the Penis

Man, for better or worse, has the largest penis of all primates.

••••••••••••••••••••

THE PURPOSE OF ANY penis is to deposit sperm somewhere in the vicinity of ripe female eggs. What distinguishes man from the beasts in matters sexual is his year-round enthusiasm for the sexual act, his emotional involvement with his partner, and the fact that he enjoys orgasms. The human penis is thought to have developed to its present size in order to excite the female of the species and to enhance the pleasure of the copulatory act.

■ Time for a *Latin lesson.* Popular names for male genitalia in the days of the Roman Empire had a distinctly agricultural flavor:

Testicles: *Fabae* (beans); *mala* (apples)
Penis: *Arbor* (tree); *thysus* (stalk); *radix* (root); *falx* (sickle)
Semen: *Ros* (dew)

SIZE

■ Man has the *largest penis* of all the primates. Sizes range from about 1½ inches to an astonishing claim of nearly 19 inches from a star of porno magazines appropriately named Long Dong Silver.

■ There are plenty of myths surrounding *race* and *penis size.* The most extensive survey on size was carried out by the Kinsey team in America. They found the smallest penis among whites was 1½ inches, while the smallest penis among blacks was 2¼ inches. The largest among whites was 6½ inches, among blacks 6¼ inches. The average size for whites was 4 inches, for blacks 4½ inches.

■ The size of the *male nose* is supposed to relate directly to the size of the penis.

■ The size of the *flaccid penis,* fully stretched, is the same as the measurement of the length of the erect penis.

■ In a study of 80 men—40 of whom had penises measuring 2 to 3½ inches in length and 40 whose penises measured 4 to 4½ inches— the greatest increase from flaccid to erect state occurred in the *man with the smallest penis* (his penis actually doubled in size). The most insignificant increase—under 2 inches—was recorded in a man whose penis measured 4½ inches. However, the author of the survey admits that conditions were not strictly clinical, that measurement was frequently rushed, and as a consequence, these statistics cannot be considered definitive—just interesting.

■ *Short men are sexy.* In yet another fascinating survey, this time of 312 men somewhere in America, the largest penis in the group (5½ inches) belonged to a man just 5 feet 7 inches tall.

The size of a man's penis is in no way related to body size. It is entirely a matter of *heredity.*

■ A boy's penis reaches *adult proportions* at about the age of 17.

■ The *bushmen* of the Kalahari desert have semierect penises all the time.

■ Changes in the penis during sexual excitement can be measured under laboratory conditions using a mercury-filled rubber tube, which is looped around the penis and acts as a *strain gauge.*

■ The urethra—the passage through the penis for urine and semen—increases in both length and *diameter* during sexual excitement.

INCREASING DIMENSIONS

■ The *Caramoja* tribe of northern Uganda elongate their penises by tying a weight on the end. Sometimes they get so long that the men have to literally tie a knot in them.

> 99 percent of young men and women masturbate occasionally, and the 100th conceals the truth.
> —*The Encyclopedia of Sexual Behavior,* by Havelock Ellis

■ Yes, you can have the operation. Using flaps of skin and tissue from the groin, the penis can surgically be extended. This risky procedure, which can result in a penis up to two times its original length, is undertaken only on patients with *extremely short* penises.

If you can't face the knife, try chapter 2 of the *Kama Sutra,* in which you will be advised to rub the member before copulation with tepid water and then anoint it with honey and ginger. This may *sting* and will certainly be *sticky.*

For cures more desperate than the affliction, we turn to the Arabs, who have developed some very interesting methods of penis enlargement involving the use of hot pitch, bruised leeches, and boiled asses' penises. Such desperate measures should be *avoided.*

If all else fails, the *Kama Sutra* claims that an ointment made of the fruit of the koklaksh, whatever that may be, will contract the yoni of an elephant woman for *one night.*

MUTILATION

Many peoples of the world feel they have to improve on nature with surgery.

■ *Australian aboriginals* have been known to slit the penis through to the urethra so that it can be flattened out to resemble the forked penis of the kangaroo.

■ The *Peguans* of south Burma used to insert little gold and silver bells under the skin of the penis.

■ The *Dayaks* of Borneo insert, across the top of the penis, a metal rod with balls fixed to the ends. Rich Dayaks use golden balls, poor ones use pebbles.

■ In some African tribes, only the chief's eldest son was allowed to procreate. To this end, all the other sons had a transverse cut made across the urethra, just in front of the scrotum. The men thus were not denied their sexual pleasure, but their semen, and come to that their urine, never made it to the tip. Amongst Europeans this operation was known colloquially as *whistle cock.*

■ In *ancient Rome,* entertainers (musicians, actors, and the like) had holes made in the foreskin and a ring inserted, presumably to stop them taking advantage of their enraptured female fans.

■ Top athletes in *ancient Greece,* it is alleged, had their foreskins tied over the top of the glans to prevent them from weakening themselves by having intercourse.

■ *Polynesians* slit the foreskin lengthwise at puberty.

■ Some tribes in *Africa* and in *Polynesia* have practiced semicastration—the removal of one testicle.

■ *Total castration,* luckily now rare, has been practiced throughout the world either as a punishment, to produce eunuchs for guard duty at temples and in harems, or to produce singers with fine high voices. Men who have been castrated before puberty retain the hair distribution, voice, and temperament of boys and are, of course, sterile. The effects on a man of castration after puberty vary according to the age and maturity of the individual, but the unfortunate victim almost always will tend to be fat.

DISPLAY AND DECORATION

■ In some parts of *New Guinea* and *Borneo* men wear no clothing at all, except for an enormously long and colorful penis sheath made from a gourd—the purpose being to draw attention to the penis, not to hide it.

■ The males of the *Mambas* tribe of the New Hebrides often wrap their penises in yard after yard of calico, winding and folding it into a neat bundle some 17¾ inches long. The purpose is to protect the wearer from the evil eye.

■ *Penis sheaths* are a popular form of attire throughout the Third World. Toothpaste tubes, discarded film containers, opened sardine cans, and even the leg of a plastic doll have been spotted fulfilling this remarkable role in parts of New Guinea and South Africa.

■ In 14th-century Europe, high-ranking noblemen were permitted to display their *naked genitals* below a short tunic—their tightly fitting hose were not joined at the crotch. If their genitals were not of sufficient size to make a fine display dangling enticingly beneath their doublets, they wore a braquette, a form-hugging padded falsie make of skin-colored leather.

> Any knight under the rank of a lord, or any other person [is forbidden to wear] any gowne, jaket, or cloke unless it be of sufficient length on a man standing upright to cover his privy member and buttokkes.
>   —Law passed in 1548 by King Edward VI

■ In the 15th and 16th centuries, European fashion favored the *codpiece.* Padded, stiffened, embroidered, bedecked with bows and sometimes with jewels, the codpiece—though it had its origins in modesty—was an explicit sexual signal. The modern double-stitched trouser fly is supposed to be the last vestige of the codpiece.

■ In English law, *indecent exposure,* which is defined as the display of the penis, flaccid or erect, toward a person of the opposite sex, is an exclusively male offense. It is the most common sexual misdemeanor.

PROTECTION

■ The *condom* was invented by an English army doctor called Colonel Condom. He made it for Charles II from a length of lamb's gut. Condoms (used for birth control and the prevention of venereal disease) were made of animal gut until the early 1840s, when a certain Mr. Goodyear discovered how to make them out of rubber.

■ The most common method of sterilization for men is *vasectomy,* in which the vas deferens (the tubes carrying the sperm) are cut. It is quick, simple, and effective. A typical survey reveals that after the operation, 74.5 percent of men experienced no difference in their sex drive, 17.9 percent experienced an increase, and a paltry 7.9 percent reported a small decrease.

SENSITIVITY

■ The human glans penis is about as sensitive as the *sole of the foot.*
·■ There is *no difference* in sensitivity between the circumcised penis and the uncircumcised one.
■ Premature ejaculation is not caused by an overly sensitive penis but by lack of emotional control. *So there.*

PROLONG THE PLEASURE

■ A few dietary tips from the *Kama Sutra* may come in handy. *Many eggs* fried in butter and then immersed in honey will make the member hard for the whole night. It may also make you *sick*.

■ *Camel's* milk mixed with honey produces surpassing vigor and causes the virile member to be on the alert night and day.

■ Take one part of the juice from pounded onions and mix with two parts of honey. Heat it over a fire until the juice disappears. Let the residue cool and preserve it. Mix one measure with three of water, and macerate chick-peas in the fluid for one day and one night. Take this beverage before going to bed, and a man will have his member rigid and upright without intermission. This should not be used three nights in succession, and *never in the summertime*.

■ If you should happen upon a *camel hump,* melt down some of the fat and rub your member with it.

■ An endorsement for the *onion* from *The Perfumed Garden:*

The member of Abou el Keiloukh
has remained
erect
For thirty days without a break
because he
did eat onions.

From *Facts and Phalluses* by Alexandra Parsons

Part 12

ASK MEN'S HEALTH

Ten Questions Men Ask Most

From nutrition to sex to hair loss—
here are the answers to the questions nearly every
guy has asked at least once in his life.
In case you haven't—it's about time you did!

● ●

MEN TODAY are faced with an enormous variety of choices and responsibilities, while society sends mixed messages about what it takes to be a "real" man. No wonder men are often confused. Here are several of the questions that men seem to be asking most often these days. The answers are based on information from top authorities in nutrition, health, and relationships.

WHAT NUTRIENTS DOES A MAN NEED MOST?

One way to answer this question is to look at nutrients known to play a role in preventing health problems to which men are particularly prone. These "male nutrients" combat cardiovascular problems, help prevent cancer of the colon, or ameliorate the increasingly common problem of infertility. They're also nutrients we are likely to neglect, given our less-than-perfect diet.

With these considerations in mind, it could well be argued that magnesium, vitamin C, zinc, and fiber (although fiber is actually a food component, not a nutrient) are some of the most important elements in a man's diet. There are dozens of ways this humble nutritional foursome can maximize a man's health. And it's not that difficult to get enough: Just stop thinking less like a man and more like a rabbit.

Magnesium (RDA: 350 milligrams/day)

This mineral plays a part in keeping your heart muscles beating rhythmically. Research suggests that too little magnesium can upset the delicate balance in the calcium, magnesium, and potassium content of the cardiac muscle cells. Imbalance increases the risk for development of cardiac arrhythmias, sudden death, ischemic heart disease (heart attacks), hypertension, transient ischemic attacks, and strokes, according to some researchers.

There's also evidence that magnesium helps keep the tiny blood components called platelets from clumping together and blocking blood vessels. It may also prevent coronary arteries from going into spasm and cutting off blood flow to the heart, which can result in the chest pains of angina or even a heart attack. The latest news about magnesium is that it may help men not only to avoid a heart attack but also to survive should one occur.

Yet most of us still don't get the magnesium we need. The body is deprived of magnesium in a number of different ways, researchers say. Boiled and steamed foods are drained of magnesium before they even enter the body. You lose magnesium through sweat when you exercise. Drinking alcohol can drain off more of the mineral. And stress greatly accelerates the loss of magnesium from the body—at the same time magnesium deficiency leads to increased stress. And as you get older, your body becomes less able to efficiently absorb magnesium from foods. Add to this the fact that older people tend to eat less food in the first place, and you have the arithmetic of magnesium deficiency.

To boost your magnesium levels, eat more seafood (particularly shrimp, clams, and crab), spinach, whole grains, peas, beans, corn, cabbage, cashews, and almonds.

Vitamin C (RDA: 60 milligrams/day)

Scurvy, the vitamin C–deficiency disease once the scourge of the British sailor, is rare these days. But today's man, especially a man who eats a high-fat diet or works near toxic materials, may still need more vitamin C than he's getting.

Vitamin C, surprisingly enough, may help prevent heart disease in several different ways. A study in India showed that vitamin C "distinctly prevented" the blood's tendency to clump together, or aggregate. (Aggregation is one of the factors responsible for the development of coronary artery disease.)

And a Scottish study found that within two months, 1 gram of vitamin C a day produced a 16 percent drop in the mean cholesterol levels of a group of healthy people, ages 24 to 34. Among a group of healthy older people (55 to 61 years), vitamin C lowered mean cholesterol levels 14 percent, but more slowly—it took 6 to 12 months, according to a report in the *Scottish Medical Journal*.

Good food sources of vitamin C include citrus fruits, green peppers, papayas, brussels sprouts, broccoli, cantaloupes, cauliflower, and strawberries.

Zinc (RDA: 15 milligrams/day)

Male sexual maturity and fertility depend on adequate zinc, which the body needs to make protein. Zinc-containing enzymes help string together the long chains of amino acids that make up each molecule of protein. And every cell's genetic material, its DNA and RNA, is derived from protein. Because of its role in DNA and protein synthesis, a deficiency may "adversely affect cell division and restrict testicular growth," says Ananda Prasad, M.D., of Wayne State University School of Medicine.

Zinc also exerts a profound influence on the body's ability to resist disease. There's also evidence that zinc can prevent toxic metals like cadmium and lead from accumulating in the body.

Foods high in zinc include seafood, liver, mushrooms, sunflower seeds, soybeans, and brewer's yeast.

Fiber (Recommended: 30 grams/day)

More salad, beans, peas, fruit, and whole-wheat bread are exactly what we need. Plant foods are the richest source of fiber— that indigestible "bulk" or "roughage" that passes right through the body without yielding to gastric acids. And although fiber by itself does not provide nutrients, it greatly affects the way the body absorbs them and is as important to good health as any mineral or vitamin.

Low-fiber diets have been linked to colon cancer, coronary heart disease, diabetes, obesity, and high blood pressure. That's a good part of the whole miserable catalog of Western man's health complaints.

There are five different types of fiber—cellulose, hemicellulose, mucilage, pectin, and lignin—each with its own special benefits. For men, water-soluble fiber like mucilage and pectin is of particular interest, because it can help clear the blood of artery-clogging cholesterol.

Oatmeal is a good source of mucilage—almost one-half the bulk of rolled oats is water-soluble fiber, and studies show oat bran can lower serum cholesterol levels significantly. A fiber-rich diet also can selectively reduce levels of LDL cholesterol (low-density lipoproteins, often referred to as "the bad kind") and raise levels of HDL cholesterol (high-density lipoproteins, "the good kind").

Pectin is another water-soluble fiber that appears to have some cholesterol-lowering abilities. Apples, oranges, pears, carrots, and beets contain pectin.

Probably the most serious consequence of a fiber-depleted diet is the increased risk of developing colon cancer, the second most common kind of fatal cancer in men. It's thought that fiber may protect the colon by speeding up the passage of cancer-causing substances through the intestine. The class of hemicellulose fiber called the *pentosans* may prove protective against colon cancer. Pentosan fiber can be found in berries, bananas, and plums and in common vegetables like cauliflower, broccoli, potatoes, spinach, and eggplant.

Some high-fiber foods may help control diabetes by slowing down the body's absorption of sugar after a meal. Compared with highly refined foods, fiber-rich foods give a feeling of fullness more quickly, making it easier to eat less and thus helping combat obesity, a health hazard of major proportions. Experts suggest a fiber intake of 30 grams a day.

WHAT ARE THE BEST FOODS I CAN EAT?

Some of the most traditional masculine meals are also the most nutritionally high-powered. Here's a look at the healthful benefits of five manly food groups.

Hunter Foods

Hunting is in our blood. But so is cholesterol. And fat. Too much of both.

But if we're born to hunt, how can meat be so harmful to the male heart? Didn't we thrive on the stuff for centuries before the red in red meat began to say "Stop!"?

Meat's not the problem; it's how we get it. Beef bred for the table is like no animal that ever lived before. Confined and fed high-energy rations, beef cattle put on body fat at a rate impossible to achieve in the wild.

Slap your average beefsteak on a grill, and you're looking at a slab of meat that's about 30 percent fat. Trim every last visible scrap from it, and you're down to 15 or 18 percent. Sounds good, until you realize that wild game like deer, moose, and caribou averages only 2 to 4 percent fat!

Some breeders are now coming up with super-lean beef. Look for more of this healthier beef to come on the market, along with ranch-raised venison.

Meanwhile, enjoy the leaner cuts of beef (trimmed of white stuff) already available: bottom round, eye of round, sirloin, and flank steak (also known as London broil).

Gatherer Foods

Early man was a hunter, yes, but that was only half the story— our ancestors were actually hunter-gatherers. Today, science tells us that the vegetal foods our ancestors gathered play an important role in good health. Plant foods can actually help protect man against heart disease and cancer of the lungs, bowel, and prostate. Here's why:

■ Vegetables and fruits have no cholesterol.
■ They contain almost no fat, and the little they do have is of a beneficial nature.

■ They're full of fiber, which is probably good for both your heart and digestive tract.

■ The green leafies and most fruits and vegetables that have a red or orange color are packed with beta-carotene, a form of vitamin A that most scientists now feel helps protect against a number of different cancers. Look for spinach, kale, broccoli, carrots, squash, pumpkin, sweet potatoes, peaches, and apricots—all super sources of beta-carotene, plus the other health bonuses of gatherer foods.

Fisherman Foods

Medical scientists say that any man thinking insurance for his heart ought to be thinking fish. Doctors have discovered that the form of fish oil found plentifully in cold-water fish like tuna, mackerel, herring, salmon, and trout has something about it that can lower harmful blood fats, help relieve painful angina of the coronary vessels, and make your blood less likely to form an abnormal clot that could produce a heart attack or stroke.

The oils belong to a group known as omega-3, and someday omega-3 may gain the status of a powerful natural preventive medicine. All fish have some of this apparently protective oil, and all are also low in harmful saturated fats.

Cowboy Foods

Beans, pardner. Of all the high-fiber foods that scour cholesterol from the system, probably none is more effective than beans. The particular form of fiber found in beans is especially valuable to begin with, and beans are a food you can eat in goodly amounts.

Lentils and navy, pinto, red, black, white, soy, garbanzo (chickpeas), and fava beans are the prime providers of bean power. If they tend to overpower you, here's a tip: Soak the beans overnight. Using fresh water, cook them for ½ hour; then discard the cooking water, replace it with fresh water, and cook until the beans are tender.

Fire Foods

For socially objectionable foods that are polite to your innards, consider these three fire breathers: garlic, onions, and hot peppers.

Although it may sound like folklore, many medical studies have confirmed that garlic and onions have the potency to knock down blood fats just like fish oils and beans do, though through a different mechanism. It takes a certain amount of dedication, if not recklessness, to eat enough garlic and onions to do a major crunch job on cholesterol. Still, every bit helps.

As for red hot peppers, only one study's been done—in Thailand—but it revealed an unsuspected fact about the fiery cuisine of southeast Asia. What the peppers do, research showed, is temporarily "thin" the blood. That is, they reduce the likelihood of a blood clot—perhaps interrupting the kind of abnormal clotting that can lead to a stroke or thrombosis. The researchers speculate that someone who, like the Thais, eats hot peppers several times a day may be conducting a regular kind of coronary housecleaning operation.

All sort of theoretical, but a good enough excuse to douse your lean meat, fish, and beans with all the savory spices your heart desires.

CAN I LOWER MY BLOOD PRESSURE THROUGH DIET?

Yes, you can, says Cleaves Bennett, M.D., medical director of the Los Angeles InnerHealth Clinic and coauthor of *The Control Your High Blood Pressure Cookbook.* So what items do Dr. Bennett and others put on their patients' shopping lists, and why? Here are their suggestions.

Much Ado about Magnesium

"Magnesium is probably one of the most promising and least-used minerals when it comes to blood pressure control," says Burton Altura, M.D., Ph.D., a leading researcher. In studies, magnesium shows a strong link between high intake and low blood pressure.

Stock up on beans and nuts to guarantee that you'll get plenty of magnesium. Whole grains, leafy greens (like beet greens and Swiss chard), and many other fruits and vegetables are also good sources. Hard water can be a good source of many minerals, including magnesium.

The Calcium Connection

Only recently have researchers noted that some cheese and milk lovers seem to have lower blood pressure. Now they are pinpointing just who benefits from additional calcium.

"Additional calcium seems to work best for people who are hypertensive and salt-sensitive," says Lawrence Resnick, M.D., of the Cardiovascular Center at New York Hospital–Cornell Medical Center. Studies indicate that the more salt elevates blood pressure, the more calcium lowers it. Calcium, it seems, may be a way for some people to have their salt—at least in moderation—and lower their blood pressure, too.

Low-fat dairy products are excellent choices for calcium. Other good calcium sources are sardines, salmon, leafy greens, and nuts.

Pick Up on Potassium

People already taking blood pressure medicines know their doctors keep a careful watch on their potassium levels. Some drugs make the body excrete potassium. But giving extra potassium to people with mildly elevated blood pressure can make pressure drop, sometimes dramatically, according to recent studies.

Good Fat, Bad Fat

Butter, oil, bacon—all the fats we eat affect blood pressure, because they are used by the body to make hormones known as *prostaglandins*. Some prostaglandins lower blood pressure, and whether the body manufactures this kind depends on which "building materials" it has on hand.

There are two important things to remember when you're changing the fat content of your diet to try to lower your blood pressure. First, keep your total fat intake low—ideally, less than 30 percent of your total calories. Cut back on butter, margarine, oils, hard cheeses, fatty meats, and other concentrated fat sources. Second, get more than half your fat as polyunsaturates, monounsaturates, and omega-3 fatty acids. All these fats appear to have blood pressure–lowering effects.

Avoid Alcohol Altogether

Heavy drinkers have much higher blood pressure than those who drink less. And an Australian study has shown that even moderate drinking can cause blood pressure to rise.

Lose Some Weight

Finally, if you could use some inspiration to lose weight, consider this: Losing weight is sometimes the only thing people need to do to drop their blood pressure to normal.

And you don't necessarily have to lose it all! Losing even one-third or one-half of your excess weight can have a tremendous impact on your blood pressure, Dr. Cleaves Bennett says. Luckily, the same foods that help your blood pressure in other ways can help you lose weight, too.

IS WALKING GOOD ENOUGH TO DELIVER FITNESS?

A vigorous walking program delivers many of the same benefits as jogging but with far less chance of injury to joints, bones, or tendons, and it improves heart/lung fitness. Regular distance walking may also improve your blood fat profile by reducing cholesterol and triglycerides, cutting down blood pressure, and lowering body weight and fat stores. Reductions in body fat, cholesterol, and blood pressure lower your risk of heart disease.

But Is It Demanding Enough?

Dyed-in-the-wool runners may find it hard to believe that walking is actually demanding enough to do you any good, but regular walking ranks right up there with other aerobic sports.

For most adults, fast walking may indeed offer an adequate aerobic training stimulus. But it's not necessary to walk at maximum speed to benefit from walking. In fact, devotees of the boardwalk stroll will be happy to know that even walking at slow speeds increases your metabolism.

And you burn about the same number of calories *per mile* if you walk at a 2-, 3-, or 3½-mile-per-hour pace. Walking 5 miles an hour (close to top walking speed) produces about the same energy expenditure as slow jogging. And if you're racewalking—doing 6 or 7 miles an hour—you may actually be expending *more* calories than a jogger.

There's something else to be said for walkers who don't want to get anywhere fast. A program of regular physical activity is more beneficial than a vigorous training program to improve short-term conditioning. In other words, whatever exercise you pick, do it regularly. And that's one of the great things about walking: It's inherently pleasant, so it's easy to keep on doing.

The Walking Prescription

How much would a healthy middle-aged man have to walk in order to stay in condition? As a general rule, says Barry Franklin, Ph.D., director of the Cardiac Rehabilitation and Exercise Laboratories at William Beaumont Hospital in Royal Oak, Michigan, 30 minutes of brisk walking, three times a week, would be a minimum program for adult men. An optimal program: 45 to 60 minutes, four times a week. (By "brisk," Dr. Franklin means a pace of about 3½ to 4½ miles per hour.)

You have to keep the total "energy cost" of your walks sufficiently high. To do that, you can adjust any one of the three most important variables of exercise to suit yourself: intensity, duration, or frequency. "If you don't want to increase your pace, for instance, all you have to do is walk a little farther or walk a little more often," Dr. Franklin says.

A 155-pound man burns about 80 calories walking 1 mile at anywhere from 1 to 4 miles an hour, he says. You'd burn around 120 calories if you ran that mile. So if you just walk 1½ miles, you'll burn as many calories as if you'd run 1 mile.

WILL EXERCISE OR DIET HELP ME LOSE MORE WEIGHT?

Given the choice, men will usually choose exercising more rather than eating less as a way to lose weight. But which road is the wiser to travel?

"If you could choose only one, probably exercise," says Michael Lowe, Ph.D., director of Temple University's weight management program. "Dieting without exercise risks loss of muscle tissue, and a would-be weight loser certainly doesn't want that."

Research indicates, too, that weight loss via exercise results in more favorable changes in blood fats: HDLs (those heart-helping high-density lipoproteins) get a boost, while LDLs (villainous low-density lipoproteins) get a boot. Dieting without exercise usually results in decreases in HDL and LDL alike.

And keep in mind that eating better—notice we didn't say eating less—can facilitate a weight-loss program immensely. "The key to making weight loss as healthful and as easy as possible is to get diet and exercise working in tandem," Dr. Lowe says. "Fat will be lost faster, muscle tissue will be spared, and health will be optimally enhanced."

So here we go: dieting tips best suited for getting that fat-burning tandem in gear.

Don't go on a diet—fix the one you have. The biggest mistake most men make in dieting is that they bite off more than they can chew. When you make a dietary change, ask yourself whether you'll be able to keep with it for the next ten years. If not, it may be too extreme. It's better to gradually ease into a more healthful style of eating than to try to become a convert overnight.

Remember that the longer weight loss takes, the longer it's apt to last. You shouldn't try to lose weight faster than about 1 percent of your existing body weight per week. For a 200-pounder, that's no more than 2 pounds a week. Go any faster than that, and you risk more than making yourself miserable—your body could flip into what weight-loss experts call the "starvation response," where the body conserves fat as it would during a famine.

Consider dietary fat your worst enemy. Fat not only beats protein and carbohydrates in the calorie department (fat contains 9 calories per gram, compared with about 4 for carbos and protein) but also is a proven no-no for the heart. And it's downright eager to turn into flab: Only one-fifth as much energy is required to convert dietary fat into body fat as is required for carbohydrates.

Consider dietary fiber your best friend. High-fiber foods are more than filling: Research suggests that fiber may actually help erase calories from other foods by sweeping them through the intestines before they've had a chance to be digested. Studies show, too, that certain types of fiber are effective at lowering blood fats and blood pressure and reducing the risk of colon cancer.

Throw away your scale. Or at least hide it. Frequent weighings can confuse a weight-loss campaign by showing temporary fluctuations such as water retention or positive situations such as muscle gain. Simply looking in a mirror or keeping track of your waist size can tell you more about your progress than any scale.

Count satisfaction, not just calories. Keeping satisfied is important not just for avoiding binges but also for keeping weight loss working metabolically. The body reacts to extreme hunger by putting the brakes on calorie burning—so pull calories from your diet in ways your body is least likely to notice. Try a leaner cut of steak or light beer instead of the real thing.

Be realistic about alcohol. Alcohol's calories may not be the fat-producing equivalent of the calories in food, but alcohol has other effects that can make it fattening, as anyone who's ever gone through an entire pepperoni pizza after a night of merrymaking can sadly attest.

Expect plateaus. They're a natural part of the weight-loss process and should not be cause of disillusionment or concern. Weight loss will resume as soon as the body has had a chance to make certain necessary metabolic adjustments.

Don't seesaw. It's okay and perhaps even advisable to take occasional vacations from a weight-loss effort—periods where you maintain rather than continue to lose—but don't backslide. Research now shows that weight loss may get more difficult each time you do it, so do yourself the favor of doing it just once.

WHAT CAN I DO ABOUT MY THINNING HAIR?

You can lose loads of hair before anyone notices and before the basic look of your hair changes dramatically. During the first years of male pattern baldness—perhaps for as long as eight or ten years—you can keep the look of your hair intact by making the hair you have look thicker. Here's how, according to George Roberson, Manhattan hairstylist and author of the book *Men's Hair.*

Shampoo frequently. If your hair is oily, it is heavy and sticks together, making it look thin. Frequent shampooing (every day if necessary) removes excess oil and gives hair a fuller look.

Use conditioners. Many hair conditioners coat hair shafts, giving each shaft some extra thickness.

Try moving your part. After a shower, pat—don't rub—your hair dry. While your hair is damp, try wearing it with a different part. Your hair will automatically have more lift because you're changing the root direction of the hair. Just lowering or raising your part can make your receding hairline unnoticeable.

Avoid the plastered-down look! Sweeping long side hair up and over a balding top doesn't fool anyone. Just tousling your hair and not wearing a definite part will make your hair look thicker. Moving your hair with spread fingers will give the hair direction, and you'll get more lift.

Cut your hair shorter overall. If you have a large, horseshoe-shaped bald spot on the top of your head, you have two options. Cut your hair relatively close to the head, so it is in proportion with your face (from ½ inch to 1 inch). Your hair will then look neat and natural. Your other option is to replace the hair you've lost.

Keep all your hair in proportion. Don't grow long hair on the back and sides of your head if the hair is thinning on top. It's much better to keep all your hair in proportion, because longer hair lies flat and limp under its own weight. The longer hair is, the more it weighs. Shorter hair always has more lift.

Use less creme rinse. Creme rinses can weigh the hair down. If you use only a dot, a dime-sized dollop, your hair will get the benefits of the creme rinse (shine, manageability) without the heaviness.

Change your hair groomer. If you're using one of the oily-type groomers, such as Oily VO5, Brylcreem, or Clairol's Vita-point, switch to a nonoily groomer, such as Dep, Tenax, Clinique's Hair Shaper, or Aramis Multiplexx.

Try blow-drying with a setting lotion. When hair is damp, lift up half-inch sections and spray the setting lotion on the roots of the hair. Just spray the areas where you want more lift (usually the top). Use the blow dryer on medium heat. With one hand holding the dryer at least 10 inches from your head, use the other hand to pull the hair upward lightly as you aim the air from the dryer at the roots of the hair.

Get a color rinse. You'll need a professional's help for this technique, but it may well be worth it. Color rinses don't necessarily change the color of your hair. They do, however, add body and lots of shine, which is just the right prescription for thinning hair.

Lighten your hair. For men with dark, thinning hair, the color difference between their hair and scalp is intense, magnifying the lack of hair density. By lightening your dark hair just a few discreet shades, you can eliminate the strong contrast. Thinning hair becomes denser looking.

Try some diversionary tactics. Beards and moustaches do this. A flattering, sculpted bit of facial hair draws attention away from your head, focusing it down onto your face.

Get a body wave. A body wave is an easy way to give more fullness to the hair on top of your head. Your hairstylist may wave only the hair on top of your head and then blend it more easily with the bulkier hair on the sides and back, or you could have a full body wave to make all the hair on your head thicker. The hair is then cut shorter on the sides and back to give it the look of overall equal proportions.

Stop worrying about your hair. So you're losing it. So what? Haven't you got a personality? A career? A good brain? A nice smile? It could be that you have been so preoccupied with your receding hair that you've been ignoring your good points.

Sean Connery goes on television shows all the time without his toupee. He's happy, healthy, and wears the hairpiece only in the movies. He's obviously not ashamed to go in public au naturel.

If you're losing your hair, start shaping up the rest of you. If a well-dressed man with a beautifully fit body comes into a room, looking happy and healthy, the last thing anybody is going to notice about him is whether he has a bald spot.

SHOULD I CONSIDER PLASTIC SURGERY?

Yes, says Mary Ruth Wright, Ph.D., a clinical assistant professor of psychology at Baylor College of Medicine in Houston, "if you want physical rather than psychological results. Cosmetic surgery does not change personality—it changes appearance." Dr. Wright is quite specific about about who *shouldn't* have cosmetic surgery: "Individuals with low self-esteem, a long history of inadequacies in personal, sexual, and working relationships, and vagueness about what they want. A man who won't face natural aging. A man who is in a crisis situation. A man who has unresolved grief—anyone who is in a depression or a grief period does not have the emotional reserve to go through elective surgery. Another problem is a man who focuses everything on a single, physical defect—for example, a man who blames all his disappointments on his large nose."

Does Your Surgeon Get under Your Skin?

"It's very important for the patient to feel comfortable with his doctor," says John Goin, M.D., clinical professor of surgery at the University of Southern California School of Medicine and coauthor of *Changing The Body: Psychological Effects of Plastic Surgery.* "The relationship between the cosmetic surgeon and the patient, while time-limited, is a close relationship. Not liking a particular surgeon is a good reason to find another."

Dr. Goin says that for best results, you should also feel confident about your surgeon's abilities. "Ask your primary-care doctor— an internist or a family practitioner—for a recommendation. A family practitioner has usually seen the work of many plastic surgeons. He knows who's overcharging, and who does good work from a technical standpoint, and who rejects patients for cosmetic surgery from time to time—which is a very good sign.

"Another hallmark of competence is board certification in plastic surgery. Not all doctors who perform plastic surgery are board-certified in this specialty. Fellowship in the American College of Surgeons is a good sign—this group is very concerned about ethics and investigates candidates for membership."

Fear from Ear to Ear

"My experience is that the more overtly worried the patient is, the better he tends to do," says Dr. Goin. "Male patients have a tendency to bottle their anxiety up a bit. They feel it isn't appropriate for a man to express a lot of fear. Because of this, they sometimes have a rougher time tolerating pain and disfigurement after surgery."

Wait a minute—did that doctor say there's *disfigurement* after surgery?

"One of the most important things that people need to realize about cosmetic surgery is that they'll look *worse* before they look better," says Dr. Goin. "We're the only specialty that takes well people and makes them sick. You'll be bruised. You'll be swollen. You'll hurt." Knowing that these changes will take place after surgery— and that they're temporary—is the best psychological preparation.

Nine Slices of Life

Here's the lowdown on the most commonly performed types of cosmetic surgery. The numbers below are based on operations performed in 1986 by members of the American Society of Plastic and Reconstructive Surgeons.

Nose surgery (rhinoplasty). *Number performed on men: 20,558; percentage performed on men: 25 percent.* Whether a nose is bent, bumpy, or big, the operation is basically the same. You're sedated and given a local or general anesthetic (standard for all cosmetic surgery). The surgeon goes in through the nostrils and makes incisions inside the nose, which is why there's no visible scar. He separates skin from bones and goes to work. If it's a bump, he saws it away and brings the nasal bones together to make a narrower bridge. If a new tip is what's wanted, he removes cartilage and reshapes. For a smaller nose, the bones are chiseled into shape.

Eyelid surgery (blepharoplasty). *Number performed on men: 15,244; percentage performed on men: 18 percent.* This is really a fat removal operation: The surgeon makes incisions under and over the eyes and removes the fat pads. This gets rid of bags under your eyes and folds of skin over them.

Dermabrasion. *Number performed on men: 7,096; percentage performed on men: 27 percent.* Sophisticated sand papering to remove scars. The skin (derma) is abraded off, and new, smoother skin grows back. The technique can't be used to remove your old girlfriend's name from your arm. It's also not a treatment for active acne—but it can help smooth and even acne-scarred skin.

Face-lift. *Number performed on men: 6,693; percentage performed on men: 10 percent.* The C-shaped incision around the front of each ear cuts from your hairline to the back of your neck. The skin is pulled off the muscles and bones and lifted back, and the excess skin is cut off. Another incision is made under your chin, and the fat there is removed.

Ear surgery (otoplasty). *Number performed on men: 6,547; percentage performed on men: 44 percent.* Most men have this operation because of ears that don't have normal folds and so appear bowl-shaped and prominent. For this problem, the surgeon makes an incision behind the ears, weakens the cartilage, and puts in stitches so that the ear folds properly. Other operations correct protruding ears, ears that fold at the top, pointy ears—and any other strange shape you can imagine.

Body fat reduction (lipectomy). *Number performed on men: 5,966; percentage performed on men: 6 percent.* This is like maid service for your fat: The surgeon vacuums the areas you didn't have the time or energy to clean up yourself—thighs, abdomen, buttocks, you name it. The vacuum in this case is a *cannula,* a thin tube that's inserted through an incision and sucks out the fat.

Chin augmentation (mentoplasty). *Number performed on men: 2,759; percentage performed on men: 18 percent.* This surgery corrects protruding or receding chins. Working from inside the mouth, the surgeon cuts through the bone and moves the chin, wiring it into its desired position. In the case of a receding chin, he may put in a plastic implant.

Hair transplant. *Number performed on men: 2,800; percentage performed on men: 95 percent.* A surgeon can remove plugs of hair follicles and transplant them in receded areas. Or he can operate on the entire scalp, slicing it open and pulling it over so that the areas on the sides where hair still grows are now on the top.

Abdominoplasty. *Number performed on men: 2,264; percentage performed on men: 7 percent.* Usually called a "tummy tuck," this gets rid of flabby stomach muscles and loose abdominal skin. The surgeon makes an incision from hip bone to hip bone, lifts the skin, tightens the abdominal muscles and tissue with sutures, pulls down the skin and cuts off the excess, and closes the incision. Somewhere in there, he builds a new belly button, too.

ARE THERE ANY SEX SECRETS WOMEN WISH MEN KNEW?

Yes, and based on an informal survey at a mid-sized East Coast publishing company, this is the good news: Women don't want you to prove yourself—they want you to enjoy yourself! They want more leisurely, sensual, intimate lovemaking, not a goal-oriented performance. So tales of sexual prowess that impress men in the barroom aren't necessarily the same things that wow women in the bedroom. Here are the findings.

Don't worry about "The Big O." "I really wish that men weren't so hung up on female orgasm," said one woman. "The intimacy, closeness, and sharing during lovemaking can certainly be satisfying enough. Sure, orgasms are terrific, but they're not the only thing."

Said another, "I guess men are not sure how to make love without orgasm as a goal. They can't accept sexual play as satisfying in itself."

Move less, mean more. "The standard macho man's idea is to penetrate the woman and hump like a piston or a jackrabbit without missing a beat. But women want more variation. Try a circular motion. Sometimes go slow, and sometimes go fast. Women need teasing and tantalizing," says Diane Dunlap, director of the Center for Social and Sensory Learning in Los Angeles.

Her advice was echoed by the women in the survey. "Teasing your way to orgasm is the only way to go," said one woman. "Devote some time," advised another. "Instant gratification can be had easily without a partner. Why not make the most of a twosome?"

Practice basic hygiene. The two-day beard growth, B.O., and salami breath just don't make it. "A shower and a clean shave go a long way toward enhancing sexual interest," said one woman. "No caveman stuff for me," agreed another.

Help her tell you what she likes. Many women are still too shy to talk about their sexual wishes, or they're afraid of bruising the famous male ego. How can you encourage a women to tell you what she likes?

"'What do you like, baby?' is not enough," says Dunlap. Say "I like it when my chest hairs are tickled. What do you like?"

Take turns being the aggressor. Many women confessed that they would like to be more aggressive, but they're too shy or too uncertain whether their actions would be well received. "I would like to initiate more often, but I'm shy about it," says one woman. "I guess I'd rather be sure he wants me."

So take turns with "his" and "her" nights, suggests Lonnie Barbach, Ph.D., of the Psychiatry Department at the University of California Medical School in San Francisco. "Neither one of you really wants there to be just an aggressive person and a passive person," says Dunlap.

Discover the whole body. "It was wonderful when you guys discovered the clitoris," one woman said. "So now discover the rest of the body."

"Most women need clitoral stimulation, but they don't want it until later on," said Dr. Barbach. "They don't want the man to start out there."

Hands and arms and ankles are erogenous zones. So are necks, feet, legs, breasts—the whole body, in fact. Try different strokes. Alternate deep, massagelike motions with light, feathery touches. Kiss, cuddle, and caress her. Then go for the "love button."

Get off the "size" trip. "Bigger is not necessarily better when it comes to penis size," one woman stated boldly. "Too big, and it starts to irritate after too many ins and outs. I wish men would get off the size-inadequacy trip."

The sentiment was endorsed by other women. "For those who are well endowed, learn not to inflict pain," one woman advised.

Make her feel special. "Women are most satisfied with sex when they feel valued and loved," says Rosalie Chapman, Ph.D., psychologist at Scripps Memorial Hospital in La Jolla, California. "In fact, one of the main causes of lack of sexual desire is resentment. If a woman feels a man is dominating, making rules, and not listening, she'll withdraw sexually. It's her ultimate power."

"If a man doesn't talk lovingly to a woman during sex, she may feel he is using her," Dr. Chapman says.

Reassure her, too. "Even women with wonderful bodies need a whole lot of support and compliments," says Dr. Barbach. "Women are very concerned about physical appearance in our culture. Tell her she's attractive."

And be specific. "One of my best memories is someone telling me I had sexy hair when it fell across his shoulders or how firm my body was to touch," said one woman.

"Continue to court your spouse for the rest of your life," Dr. Barbach says. "Bring her little gifts and cards. Buy her sexy lingerie. Call her on the telephone." These simple acts can help revive a relationship. What's more, they're top turn-ons, according to our survey.

Enjoy yourself. "If you try things just to give a woman an orgasm, you'll find it's getting to be work, and work doesn't work for sex," says Dr. Barbach. To please your mate, you have to please yourself. "It sounds paradoxical, but it's true," said Dunlap. "It's like comedy. Have you ever seen a green stand-up comedian? He's miserable up there, and he's frantically trying to get the audience to laugh. It's horrible for the audience to watch. . . . I don't teach men techniques in sex therapy," Dunlap said. "They start moving like machines and working for a payoff, and it never works."

"Relax and enjoy yourself," Dr. Barbach adds. "That way you'll have more interest, desire, and passion." And so will she.

WHAT'S MY KISSING MISSING?

If you've wondered whether you're remembered or quickly forgotten because of your kisses, the results of our informal poll may help. We asked a handful of ladies to critique a man's kiss and suggest how it could be improved. First, a description of the worst offenders.

The G-Man. This guy is more tight-lipped than a federal bureaucrat and just about as exciting. "Lips should be loose when you kiss, slightly puckered so they are tender when they touch. Too many men clamp their lips together when they kiss. You can feel the tension. But loose lips sink inhibitions."

The Dentist. He's determined to use his tongue to examine your molars and then wipe your tonsils for good measure. "Suffocation may be a serious side effect of being involved with this guy. A little tongue is nice, but not when it's rammed in. Use it sparingly, as a tease. Use the tip of your tongue, which is the sexy part."

The Puppy. Like man's best friend, he's so excited that he slobbers all over you. "You want to hit this guy with a rolled-up newspaper. Wet kisses are very sexy—but not when you have to take a shower after them. This guy needs to slow down and save the lapping for Fido, especially around the ears."

The Dead Fish. He's the yin to the Puppy's yang, a man whose kiss has the muscle tone of a 98-pound weakling. "No pressure, no inspiration. Are you sure you wouldn't rather be watching the Celtics game, dear?"

The Oral Rapist. He grinds your lips into your teeth, grabs everything he can get his hands on while you're unpleasantly distracted, and bites hard. "Passion is one thing. Assault is another."

The panel of experts adds that there is hope for the male gender. The main problem with men's kissing, they say, isn't a lack of ability. It's attitude. "Too many men consider kissing the appetizer they have to rush through to get to the main course," say panel members. "Give us the guy who is involved with the act of caressing your skin with his lips."

Kissing is a mood setter, and if you want the mood to last, make your kissing last. While some women like "long, searing kisses" and others prefer a series of quick exploratory movements, the entire panel agreed that their best sexual experiences were with men who took their time kissing them. "A guy who rushes through his kissing gives me a good indication of what's to follow."

Take note of how she reacts—and responds. Chances are good that she's giving you what she'd like to be getting. Passion is a delicate balance, falling between the Dead Fish and the Oral Rapist—but not too much on either side. Add some tenderness and a little tongue without being a Puppy or Dentist. She'll let you know when you hit the right combination.

Don't be shy to explore. "A woman's lips are very erogenous, but so are her ears, neck, the insides of her forearms, the back of her knees," says one. "And you don't have to rely solely on your lips. A gentle nibble with your teeth, some tongue, or even just your hot breath in the right place can really add a lot."

HOW DO WOMEN LIE TO MEN? AND WHAT CAN I DO ABOUT IT?

To find out how and why women lie to men, *Men's Health* polled women at a mid-sized, Middle American corporation, asking them what lies they tell men. Some of the lies told by single women on the dating circuit are amusing (to all but the two people involved). Some aren't. Some are white lies. Some aren't.

Much more disturbing, however, are some of the confessions of women who are married or in intimate relationships. They give us a peek at white lies gone awry, of women who lie rather than confront their mates with fundamental dissatisfactions.

Sexual Self-Denial

Over 30 percent of respondents mentioned or alluded to faked orgasms. One wrote that she had feigned orgasm when she first became sexually active but "later learned 'it' may not occur every time, and if it doesn't, you don't have to fib."

Another wrote: "I think many women, myself included, have lied to men about being sexually satisfied. What are they supposed to say? Explaining to someone that you aren't going to have an orgasm unless you do it yourself is difficult."

First-Date Fiascos

First dates are minefields of deceit. She may lie to impress you. She may lie because she's not impressed. But the first-date lies told by our respondents all have a common premise: A woman finds herself trapped for the evening with a total geek.

So one woman said, "No, I don't mind if we just watch TV and eat pizza." Another woman said, "Sounds like you have an important job." Some have said "How interesting!" when they really were bored silly.

Finally, when asked to go for a late drink after the movie, one said, "No, I'm tired. I think I'd better go home." She wrote, "Translation: Just get me out of here!"

What if that total geek is you? How can you learn to correct your flaws if nobody clues you in? Guys get indignant about these initial evasions. Women know that. Here's what one woman says: "Never believe a man who says he'd much rather have a polite but flat-out refusal from a woman. Being handed one, two, three excuses gives him the chance to bow out like it's *his* decision and leaves that eggshell ego more intact than a frank 'Thank you, but I'd rather not go out with you.' I consider this kind of lie (the avoidance turndown) to be a favor—more strain on me than on the man."

Whether or not it's a favor to anyone, the avoidance lie is the lingua franca of being young and single. Probably every man has been told, at one time or another, the equivalent of "Gee, I'd love to, but I've got to wash my hair that night."

Lies of Self-Denial

Once a woman begins to see a man on a steady basis, another kind of lie crops up. Judging from the responses, the common denominator of these lies is compromise. The hitch is, you don't know she's compromising. Outwardly, she accepts with alacrity your wishes or habits. Inwardly, she fumes.

Thus, one woman has found herself saying "Of course I don't mind if you and your dad watch the football game" and, to herself, "every damn one that's televised."

She's heard herself say, "Sure, I understand you need your freedom." Inside, she said, "I want to kill you."

Another woman lies and says, "No, I don't want to date other men." She's also swallowed and said, "No, I don't mind if you date other women."

Finally, one woman said, "Don't worry, you look fine." In truth, he needed a haircut and a tie.

Wedded Blitz

Sometimes the lies of compromise get carried into marriage. One woman, married for several years, wrote the following list of frequent lies:

- "I'd love to hear how your tennis match went."
- "Sure that shirt goes with that tie."
- "No, you don't need to shave."
- "I don't mind taking the old car."
- "I *like* cooking dinner."
- "It's no problem to pick that up."
- "I worked through lunch."
- "We only talked on the phone for a few minutes."
- "You did a great job on that!" (That's after I begged him for a month to do it!)
- I regularly give or have sex and "enjoy it" when I'd rather be sleeping.

She adds at the end, "Most of my lies are to keep the peace."

Indeed, male insecurity enters into much of the deceit revealed to us. Think of the classically insecure guy, a short-fused fellow with an "eggshell ego," as one of our respondents put it. Some women cave in to his warped will; some don't. But to a greater or lesser extent, insecure guys get babied—babied with lies.

The Truth Comes Out

How typical is the wife who could tick off ten frequent lies? There's no way of knowing, of course, from this very unscientific sample. But she is in the minority of the respondents. Most of the married women claim to lie to their husbands rarely, if at all.

One wife wrote, "I feel like I've gained confidence and assertiveness in my 'old age' and notice I've never lied to my husband. We tell it like it is—a sign, I believe, of a stable, healthy couple."

That, finally, is the picture that emerges from this group of women. The younger, single ones, dealing with insecure men and their own insecure selves, use lies because they're less volatile than the truth. But as all that gives way to more mature, stable relationships, lies become less useful. Indeed, they become much more dangerous. They could shatter years of accumulated trust.

Also evident, from this sample, is a general tone of unhappiness about lying. That flies in the face of the usual male myth about the deceiving woman. In reality, there may be only one thing to fear: her fear of you.

The Truth Helps

What about the opinion that women usually lie because men encourage it? Well, we do. We encourage all the pleasing little deceits between the sexes, just as men have done for eons.

We hate to think of our wives or girlfriends with another man, so we urge them to gloss over affairs of the past. And we expect our wives or girlfriends to be the chief source of emotional support—when we're most in need of ego boosts, we're least likely to inspect their contents.

In encouraging all these pleasing little lies, do we also discourage the truth? That's the danger.

The truth is, sometimes we have to ask for the truth.

Index